A WAR NURSE'S DIARY

Sketches from a Belgian Field Hospital

By an Anonymous World War 1 Nurse

Illustrated by Jack Champion

Written by an unknown British nurse in WW1 and first published in 1915 as *"A War Nurse's Diary: Sketches from a Belgian Field Hospital"*.

This edition published 2025
By Cosmic Jive Publishing
ISBN 978-1-918219-41-8

Cover design and illustrations are copyright Jack Champion, 2025

PART I

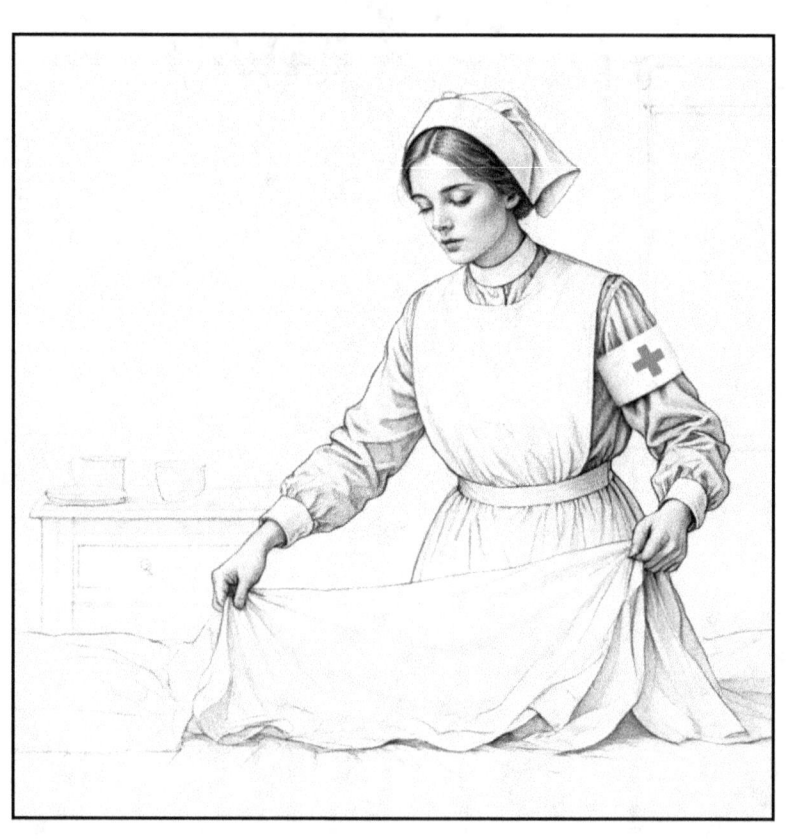

CHAPTER I
THE START

WHEN war was declared August 1st, 1914, the great upheaval sent its waves of excitement beating against every shore till it touched the whole world.

Away in the Northern-Midlands of England there is a county-hospital. Enrolled among its nurses were several who belonged to the Territorials. Scarcely had war been declared when their marching orders came. Proudly they went away, clad in military uniform, whilst those left behind envied them with an almost bitter envy.

Speaking for myself, to want a thing badly means to get it---if possible. When the Servians started I went to the Matron and asked permission to he released to offer my services. Her answer was, "Wait a little. Your own Country may need you." meanwhile she got permission for me to go. But permission to go and a zeal to serve one's country are but the preliminaries to active service at the front. Not only women but men constantly meet with bitter disappointment and many obstacles put by a wise government as tests to temper, discipline, or some inscrutable reason which like another great Power "moves in a mysterious way its wonders to perform." To make a long story short, after having filled up many forms, stating whether there was any insanity in or near the family, and what the victim's great grandmother died of, and how many foreign languages she could speak, &c., &c., &c., I was told by the Red Cross, St. John's Ambulance, the Military Nursing Reserve, and Auxiliary Bodies of many varieties, that my services were not required, as they had about thirty thousand nurses on their lists, in fact about one nurse to each soldier!

Two weeks dragged by when the post brought a correspondence card from one of our doctors with this simple legend pasted thereon;---"Ten nurses wanted at once for Antwerp; must be voluntary." Quickly I sent a wire offering my services, then waited two more interminable weeks. Having given up hope, one evening a wire was handed me, "Be ready to start to-morrow."

A lawyer came that night and helped me make a will---in case of accidents! Meanwhile my friend got two days' leave to come up with me, and next morning we were off to London.

The lady who was the organizer of our hospital had not, I should judge, any previous experience of hospitals or their management. We all felt this, and therefore were quite prepared, at an early date, to fall into the hands of the Germans, so, as a precaution, we nurses each provided ourselves with a tube of morphia tablets to take in any emergency. (They came in useful after for others, as you will see, given in smaller doses than we contemplated taking!) We were to live in tents and nurse the wounded therein. But, whatever may have been lacking in the medical arrangements, our Directress had certainly secured the names of some of the most prominent and influential people in Europe.

Our Patroness was no less a personage than Her Majesty Queen Elizabeth of the Belgians, and the Duchess de Vendôme was associated with her. Our chairman for some time was Lord Northcliffe. and afterwards Lord Sydenham, whilst many great names figured on the Committee. Our head-surgeon for some months was Mr. Souttar, F. R. C. S., one of the surgeons of the London Hospital, whilst after he returned to his work other men from the same hospital of equal repute and skill took his place.

Arriving in London we found our Directress much distressed because some of the nurses had backed out---they felt it too dangerous, I expect. Quickly I urged my friend to accept a vacancy and accompany me. She saw the Committee, was approved, and we sent the following seductive wire to her parents, "Lord------ and the Committee have accepted G------ as nurse. Please wire consent." Later on came the answer "Cannot refuse. God bless you."

We all met on Victoria Station, a motley crowd. Nine nurses in flowing violet cloaks and sky blue dresses, four or five men-doctors in khaki, three students from the London Hospital, also in khaki, four lady-doctors, three or four lay-helpers---ladies well known in society, three or four gentlemen-chauffeurs, and last, but not least, four lady farmers. These latter were dressed in officer's uniform-khaki tunic and breeches, with sun helmets. They were highly connected and highly interesting personalities. They brought with them a farm-wagon and a dray-horse, presumably because we were called a Field Ambulance! Later on we abandoned the wagon and horse, with other impedimenta.

We seemed to create a sensation at Folkestone, where we spent two nights. A film-camera operator honoured us with his attention as we marched on to the quay. Incidentally my friend sent a wire to our Matron, saying she would not be back that night, and please accept her resignation. We were casual in those days. Life seemed cheap. Matrons, whom we had hitherto looked upon as the rulers of our destinies, seemed far away in a forgotten world.

We crossed to Ostend at night. A little destroyer accompanied us, running on in front, and sometimes round and round us like a little dog out for a ran with his master. Occasionally I wondered if it was a German submarine.

Our reception at Ostend was not inspiring. We were turned out before dawn in the wet on to a large glass-covered station; the place was quite deserted and traffic was suspended. We all huddled into a waiting room; there we lived for two days and nights, placing the red plush cushions from the train-cars on the floor, where we all slept, doctors, nurses and chauffeurs. There we waited for the summons of Her Majesty the Queen of the Belgians. After two days her message came to proceed to Antwerp, where she had prepared for us a building as a hospital.

That night a train went to Antwerp with part of our staff; we watched them go out into the dark, wondering whether out of the night one of those wandering bands of Uhlans would suddenly spring upon them and wipe them out. Next morning the rest of our party embarked in our five motor cars. Along the flat roads of Northern Flanders we rushed, past Zeebrugge and Bruges and many little villages. At each place the inhabitants came out and waved their caps and handkerchiefs, shouting "Vive les Anglais!" And we shouted back "Vive les Belges et à bas les Allemands!" The whole journey was one great ovation. My first sight of the serious part of war was at a little town Ecloo leading to Ghent. There I saw a broad phalanx of soldiers clad in long, dark blue overcoats, marching grimly and sternly along. No music led them, but on they came with set faces, looking as though they would bear down and crush all before them, determination written on every countenance.

Upon entering one of the great squares of Antwerp the citizens stopped us, brought out wine and sandwiches, and insisted upon pushing our cars themselves, shouting with delight, "The English have come!".

CHAPTER II
ANTWERP

ON the Boulevard Leopold a fine building had been placed at our disposal; formerly it was a Duke's Palace, and recently a grammar school. Quickly we installed ourselves, and for the next three days our hands were full unpacking crates and getting all into working order. Scarcely had we finished when a perfect avalanche of wounded arrived, one hundred and seventy in all, more than we had beds for. We nurses turned out of our bed-room, but even then we had to fill the large landings with beds and stretchers. Every patient we received was seriously, if not dangerously, wounded; the operating-theatre was going all night; our nine nurses were scarcely able to keep abreast of the work, nor to direct the zealous, but often dangerous, energies of the body of lay-helpers who swarmed in from the neighbourhood. At 3 A. M. we had most of the patients' wounds dressed, and their poor mangled bodies resting in something like comfort.

Among the Belgian ladies who offered their services was a charming little Mademoiselle R------. Seeing we were without any resting-place, she called her father and he insisted on taking my friend and me to their house. Never can I repay those kind people for their hospitality. For nearly six weeks we stayed in their beautiful home as members of the family. After a while the other nurses were arranged for, but many had no sleep that night, for there was only a garret filled with desks and blackboards. Each night old M. R------ or one of his sons came to escort us home. We sat in a cosy sitting-room with the family, whilst the three sons told us all the latest news and rumours. These lads. were in the Garde, Civique, so knew all what was going on during the excitement and anxiety of the following weeks. How these five weeks passed is just a vague impression of constant work, conflicting rumours, rush and weariness. I can remember nothing consecutively.

My friend and I had a large flat containing fourteen wards, with seventy patients to attend to. We had no orderlies in those days; our only help was two shiftless charwomen, who talked Flemish only. All the patients were gravely wounded; they usually required two dressings a day and some much oftener. The meals alone were a perfect nightmare to get served, as scarcely any patient could feed himself; the food consisted of stews and soups in big bowls with coarse brown bread. To add to the labour, the great landing and two flights of circular stairs at either end were white marble. For the first two weeks there were only two of us to do every thing.

The Belgian R. A. M. C. officers visited the wards each morning to send on all who could travel, then they all had to be suitably clad, and the melée of muddy, disreputable uniforms sorted out and returned to the proper owners.

Two events stand out above the daily rush. The first was a visit to Malines. In that desolated town we had a dressing-station where a small party of our doctors and students went daily to render first-aid by the trenches. Never shall I forget that journey.

It was said that Antwerp was impregnable. I was told that the city had three lines of defence; the outer commenced thirty miles away in a circle of fortified towns; Termonde and Woevre St. Catherine were two of them. Then about twelve miles away were another series of towns and villages of which Malines was one. The two former towns had fallen after fierce battles, the results of which poured into Antwerp in ambulances, bleeding, broken and mangled, for us to deal with. Malines we saw; the cathedral was still standing, badly damaged but grand and magnificent. Pieces of stained glass windows, many centuries old, lay on the ground.

From Malines to Antwerp was one vast network of defences. Everywhere were reserve trenches, miles of barbed-wire-entanglements all waiting to be electrified to electrocute the enemy; great pitfalls covered with branches of trees contained sharp stakes to pinion the cavalry as they advanced; fields of pointed stakes lay at intervals to impede the horses. Immediately outside the walls of Antwerp were broad moats, alternated by high, grass-covered earth fortresses, bristling with guns. Every road into Antwerp led over a bridge; each bridge had been mined, and by touching an electric button the whole thing would blow up; great gates pierced the walls, where sentries stood at attention.

But none of these preparations was of any use; no one had reckoned upon the siege-guns and long-distance howitzers. The city fell in flames and ruins while the enemy were still eight miles or more distant. But of that, anon.

The other event to be chronicled was the coming of Winston Churchill and his Marines. Antwerp was beginning to fear; the city was packed with the constant stream of refugees carrying their bundles, all swarming in from ruined towns and villages, whilst the distant boom of guns crept nearer and nearer, and rumours grew wilder and more terrifying. At the street-corners little girls sold newspapers, and the cheery "Metropole!" was shouted out, whilst under the leading column announcing the "Situation" we were assured that everything was serene, beautiful, splendid! Then flew from mouth to mouth the news that Winston Churchill had come. The English had come! The Marines, part of England's splendid Navy, were here! Now all was well! Poor little Germans, we could even pity them as we rested secure in the power of our Navy; they would be crushed like flies and swept back to their proper place, while we had a hit at Cologne and Berlin.

It was pitiful how the Belgians trusted the British; to them they were invincible, the protectors of the weak and fallen. Wild rumours spread---it was said that the British had issued an ultimatum to Holland, that the Scheldt was to be open for six hours to allow British men-of-war to sail up and fire across the mud banks at the Germans!!

The tale of our Marines has yet to be told; one thing I know, that every one of them was a hero. They fought as Britons should---and died. That expedition was much criticized and discussed. Such things are not in a nurse's province, but we met some of the men, Marines and Tommies, and their courage and endurance amid overwhelming difficulties make one proud to be British. Twice during those weeks all our wounded were hastily removed to the great station, whilst all the many hospitals were emptied; but after waiting several hours the poor fellows were brought back again on their stretchers, cold, hungry and suffering. Naturally, if several thousand wounded from dozens of hospitals are removed hastily, it means of necessity a general mix-up of patients. Our dear boys, in whom we had a personal interest, found themselves in a strange hospital, whilst we had many of whose medical history and treatment we knew nothing.

That reminds me of "Ragtime." I must tell you about him. His real name was de Rasquinet, but, when written hastily on a chart, it looked like ragtime, and was easier to pronounce. People who do not like medical details had better skip the next few lines, but I want people to understand how "Ragtime" suffered. He was twenty-three years old, and had wonderful brown eyes that spoke his gratitude when he was too ill to utter words. He came in with his arm broken in several places and bleeding; in his abdomen were two large wounds which had pierced the intestine in several places. He also had a great wound in the back which had smashed up one kidney. At first he was too collapsed to operate upon. Such was the nature of his wounds that his dressing and the whole of his bed had to be changed at least every two hours. Imagine rolling a man in that condition from side to side. We had very little wool, we had no mackintosh sheets, brown paper was all we had to put under him; we just had to manage with rags which the neighbours supplied.

"Ragtime" was operated on; they cut out several feet of pierced intestine, joined it together and closed up the two wounds in his abdomen. The wound in the back was untouched, as he could stand no more that day. He came back to us and we nursed him with special care, along with the other sixty-nine patients. When we dressed him he never moaned nor groaned, and always gave us his wonderful smile. Then an order came for all patients to go to the station. "Ragtime" went on a stretcher with the rest. After spending twelve hours without food or attention in that draughty place, some of them came back to us, but not "Ragtime." The lady doctor and I, who attended him, searched every hospital and made every inquiry with no result.

After three days a pitiful little note came from "Ragtime," saying he was in a huge military hospital, and begging me to visit him. Catholic Sisters were in charge, and the rules were strict; finally we saw him and others who had been dumped there. He cried and implored me not to leave him. He said his wounds had not been dressed for three days! Think of it! When we dressed him it was two-hourly, and it was most necessary. The reason for the neglect was that nuns were not allowed, so I was told, to attend to men-patients below the waist! The lady-doctor went round and pleaded with them to let us have him back, but no, they would not. So I was determined. Mademoiselle and I went round and asked for the General. He was in charge of this great hospital. 1 told him the history of the case, cried and protested with real Belgian emotion, and finally the dear old General began to think that here was real romance! He let me have "Ragtime." The lady-doctor sent her car and we got him back.

Later on we left him in a hospital in Chent. Months afterwards we had an orderly, an ex-professor from a college. Wishing to join his family at Ghent he returned under the Germans. I sent by him a letter to "Ragtime." After many weeks a letter was smuggled through to me in Flemish, telling how the orderly had traced him to a certain hospital and he was lying unconscious. This made me feel that he was dying. But after another long lapse of time another man turned up who said that "Ragtime" had just been operated on for his kidney, and had been under chloroform. A year later one of our medical students met his father in a London hospital, a wounded soldier! He said that "Ragtime" was at Liège, convalescent. After the war, I shall make it my task to trace "Ragtime" in Belgium, and find out if he is alive.

Now, all this time we became busier and busier. Not only were we nursing the Belgians, but many of our British wounded came to us---Marines and Tommies. All the time we were over-crowded and understaffed, yet with all this work every one was merry and bright. Two or three times we were able to snatch an hour off duty. We went out past the streams of refugees to the fine cafés. Here English afternoon tea was served and the patisseries, as they call their cakes, were a dream, only to he had in Belgium.

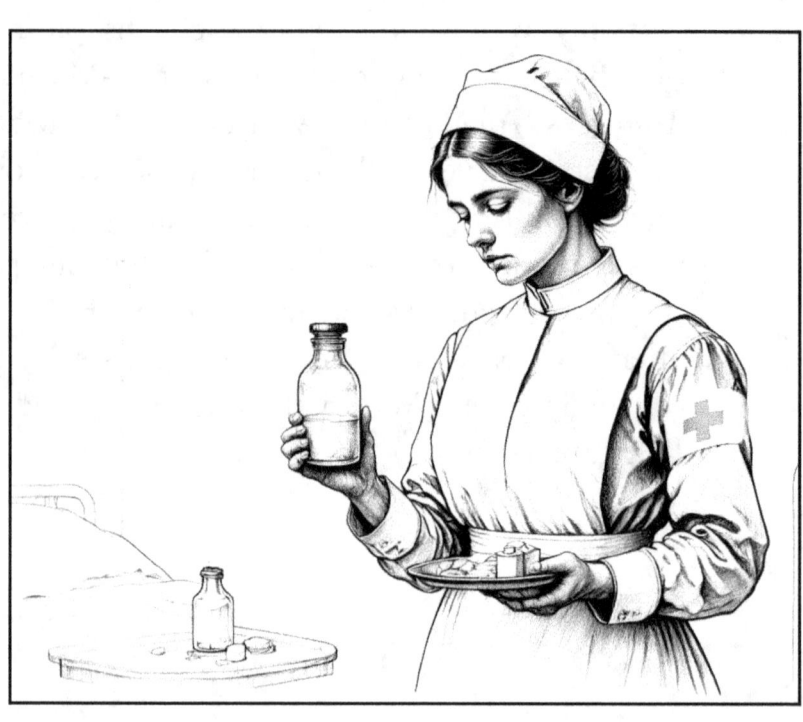

CHAPTER III
THE SIEGE

BY the end of the fourth week we had become accustomed to the constant influx of mangled and bleeding forms, and it was only upon the failure of our water supply that we clearly realized the proximity of the enemy, who was daily creeping nearer and nearer, as fort after fort fell, a mass of ruins and dead men. The Fort of Walaem witnessed a fiercely contested battle, because, not only was it an important strategic position, but there, was the reservoir which supplied the city with water. The dead British and Belgians were piled up against the walls of the reservoir, forming a ghastly barricade. The resourceful citizens immediately filled a dry-dock with the salt water of the Scheldt, purifying the water to a certain extent and connecting it with the main pipes. A notice was sent round that the taps could be used for half-an-hour each day when the supply for twenty-four hours must be drawn. Our pails and tubs were very limited, whilst our household consisted of over two hundred people, one hundred and seventy of whom were wounded men needing water in large quantities. The theatre alone used many gallons for sterilization.

As the reader perhaps knows, treating wounds in a home-hospital under surgically clean conditions is a very different thing from dealing with mangled and shattered flesh where the wounds are filled with mud, torn clothing and shrapnel. Often these men had received no first-aid treatment, and their wounds had remained uncovered for as long as two or three days. With few exceptions all these cases were septic. Our treatment for this, as a rule, was fomentations. This meant an endless supply of boiling water and constant renewal. On our floor we just placed a large tin wash-basin on a petrol stove and kept it boiling all the time. It sterilized the dressing, and the same water-supply did for every one and was always boiling. The first day we left off washing those white marble floors, the following days we stopped washing the patients, and we just kept that brackish water for medical purposes, soup and coffee.

For some days rumours were rife concerning the bombardment of Antwerp, but we did not take them seriously. It was said, truly, I believe, that all the Germans were waiting for was the setting and hardening of huge concrete foundations which they were building for their siege guns over twenty miles away.

Walaem fell five days before the bombardment of Antwerp. During that week there was a huge explosion which filled many of the hospitals in Antwerp with burnt men. Some of our wards were full of them. The injuries were confined to their faces. heads and hands, and they were often ghastly. Some were so terribly burned that it was difficult to tell where their faces were; how they lived is a marvel to us, for no features seemed left to them. We had sometimes to force an opening, where the mouth had been to insert a tube to feed them. Each man's dressing took over an hour, as even each finger had to be treated separately.

Towards the end of the first week in October a message came for all the staff to assemble in the central-hall. There our Commandant told us that the last mail boat was leaving that night, and any desirous to return to England must take the last chance. Two nurses went, and one married man.

Shortly after this another message arrived, from the Germans this time. All civilians desirous of escaping in safety must do so within the next twenty-four hours, as twenty-four hours later, at midnight, they would commence to shell the city. We never believed it, much less realized it. Already the news had spread that an Expeditionary Force was on its way to supplement the Marines and save the city. Meanwhile, things became fast and furious; there was no time to think of bombardments; it was a case of sending on all men who could possibly travel on a stretcher to make room for all who came.

Wednesday night, October 6th, as we took our usual little journey up the Boulevard to the R-----'s house, we noticed solitary figures with little bags furtively hurrying along under the cover of darkness. There was no panic; each fugitive was ashamed to leave, and still "The Metropole" proclaimed the "situation" to be serene and all well.

There was a change in the R-----'s house. All the handsome pile carpets had been rolled up and placed across the marble first floor to form a presumably bomb-proof shelter of the cellars. We went to our bedroom as usual and settled down to sleep. Our boulevard was a main road leading through one of the great city gates to the battle field. All day the roar of traffic, hoots of cars going at top speed, and lumbering of heavy lorries made a constant roar. Gradually the noise died down, whilst one heavy dray drawn by a horse rumbled over the paved street.

The city clock struck midnight, when simultaneously we heard a boom far away, immediately followed by a new whistling scream increasing in volume and intensity till it became the roar of a train in a tunnel. It skimmed over our heads, literally raising our hair in its passage. This ended in a large, full explosion. Then all was silence for a breathless second,---when the terrified roar of a wounded animal rent the air, like that of a great bull bellowing. A pistol shot followed, and silence ensued again. I was seized with an uncontrollable ague, whilst my friend reached out her hand and said, "Remember we are British women, not emotional continentals. We've got to keep our heads."

As we lay quite still in the darkness we became aware of stealthy movements outside. There was a soft knock at our door, and one of the boys said in broken English, "I sink you had better dress and come down to ze caves." We dressed and packed our holdalls, going down the back-stairs to the wine-vaults where carpets and arm-chairs had been placed. No sooner had we sat down than we realized that our place was beside our wounded. The dear old lady and gentleman urged us to stay, but after a hurried farewell, two of the sons took up our baggage and quickly escorted us to our hospital.

Twenty minutes at most had elapsed since the first shell fell. Shells were now falling at two minute intervals. Yet in that short space of time the whole of the third floor, about fifty wounded, had been quietly and methodically brought down on stretchers and placed along the network of underground passages. It was done in darkness because the roof of our house was glass. We quickly started in applying strong restoratives, after all three floors had been removed to what we deemed was safety.

About 2.00 A. M. all the patients had been settled below, with two night nurses, and the rest of us sat on some marble stairs under a colonnade until morning. As sleep was impossible, and the noise terrific, we just started singing "Tipperary," "Dixie," and other ragtime choruses to drown the explosions and buck us all up.

When morning came there was trouble in the camp. There were no servants. just one dear old woman who worked gratuitously as cook. Even she was in tears, longing to go. There was not much chance of nursing in those narrow passages, so our Chief gave me leave to help in the kitchen. Among our men were several Tommies with slight wounds; I explained the situation to them and they were fine ---full of Cockney jokes and humour. I sent them all to peel the vegetables for soup. We caught four noisy fowls who were intruders in our back yard, killed them and hung them up to the gymnasium poles to pluck. Each time a shell burst we just hopped inside, and when the pieces had scattered came out and went on with our job. We also collected the fragments of bread, for we felt we might be hungry before the end. I made four huge bread-puddings and put them in the oven. The Germans had those half baked puddings, likewise the four chickens!

I put our escape down to the German passion for system. They shelled Antwerp methodically, block by block; fortunately our section was not the object of immediate attention, only shells that fell short dropped in our locality.

At 11.00 A. M. the old cook ran out wringing her hands. "The gas has gone out," she said, for a shell had struck the gas works. This was a grave difficulty, as we had no other form of fuel. Not only could we cook no food, but the theatre, which at that moment had two tables occupied all the time, had no means of sterilizing instruments. One of our medical students had an uncle with Winston Churchill, so he just went round to Headquarters and borrowed three London Motor Omnibuses. These lumbering vehicles looked so incongruous still pasted with the latest music hall advertisements, such as "The Glad Eye," the familiar London "Elephant & Castle" marking their original destination.

It was represented to us that it was a most dangerous adventure to try to escape, but that we must save some of the more seriously wounded. Who would volunteer to attend the patients? My friend and I were standing near, so we offered. Quickly the men were packed in, as the shells fell thicker and nearer. Just at the last minute I remembered one of our patients who came in with the first batch. He was precious because he owed his life to us. When those first one hundred and seventy arrived five weeks before he was laid aside, white and pulseless, as too far gone to operate upon. We gave him restorative injections, and at last felt a feeble flutter. Running to the theatre, we begged the surgeons to give him a chance.

There was a great gash beneath his chest, and his stomach was literally lying outside of him, ripped open and covered with mud. He had been lying in that condition out on a field for two days, and according to all human calculations should have died long ago. When we asked the surgeon to operate he justly said, "We have more patients to treat than we can really get through. Those will probably live after, but it is wasting precious time to operate on your man." Finally we prevailed. They operated on him. For three days he was to have nothing by mouth, not even water. Before two days were over he had grabbed his neighbour's brown bread and bolted it greedily!

Well, this is the man I wanted to save, so I ran along to a glass house which at any minute might be wiped out by a shell, and tried to drag him along. It took some time. When we got to the front door the first convoy had gone. Standing there 1 watched a dwelling opposite, six stories high, come clattering down like a card house. The shell just went in at the roof and out at the area-grating, first exploding in the cellar. (All Antwerp was living in the cellars.) So there was not much chance for that household. Just the dismantled skeleton of the outer walls was left.

Fetching in the wounded meant constant excursions to the front door. One of the pitiful sights was the little pet dogs that came running in, looking up with pleading eyes and wagging their tails for a welcome. Just down our street, outside a closed house, from which the occupants had flown, sat a fox terrier of good breed. He was shivering with terror, but still he guarded the house whose faithless owner had forsaken him. Just then a bomb crashed near by, I whipped him up under my arm and tied him to a table leg, meaning to adopt him. We afterwards named him "Bombe."

It was now twelve noon; the Germans had cleared the town of civilians, they supposed, so they started in with howitzer shells and bombs from siege-guns. The shrapnel was child's play beside these. Instead of one house, it was now a block of buildings that went high into the air in a thick cloud of black dust and debris; when this settled down, all that remained was a mass of broken brick and dust.

The whole earth shook and it was impossible to hear people shouting. Our Chief immediately went round to that omnibus garage and commandeered five more London buses.

CHAPTER IV
THE RETREAT

WE felt in taking these buses that we were no longer robbing the Marines. Many of them were with us; many more were dead and had no use for them. It was now 3 P. M. on Thursday. As soon as the five buses arrived we commenced loading them up with our wounded. Those who could sit up were placed on top and the stretcher cases lay across from seat to seat inside. We formed a long procession, for there were five private cars as well. My car was the first to get loaded, and 1 was put in charge of the inside passengers. Shall we ever forget the loading up of those cars? They tried to save all the theatre instruments. What an eternity it seemed! Just sitting still, with the guns at last trained on to our locality.

One of the young doctors ran upstairs for his kitbag; half-way up, the wall suddenly collapsed, revealing the next house in ruins. He left that kitbag behind! Even to the last minute patients arrived, chiefly British. Just before we started a tall Marine in a navy jersey and sailor's cap was helped in. He sat in the corner next to me. All his ribs were broken down one side, and he had no plaster or support. Opposite me were two Tommies with compound fractures of the leg. 1 placed both legs on my knees to lessen the jolting.

The Marine suffered in silent agony, his lips pressed tightly together, and his white face set. 1 looked at him helplessly, and he said "Never mind me, Sister; if I swear don't take any notice." Fortunately, they had pushed in two bottles of whiskey and some soda-syphons; I just dosed them all around until it was finished. Placing the Marine's arm around my shoulders, I used my right arm as a splint to support his ribs, and so we sat for seven and a half hours without moving. Then another nurse took my place and I went up on top. During the first part of the ride I bethought me of that tube of morphia, and it came in very useful, as I gave each of those poor sufferers one or two tablets to swallow.

How can I ever describe that journey to Ghent of fourteen and a half hours? No one but those who went through it can realize it. Have you ever ridden in a London motor bus? If not, I can give little idea of what our poor men suffered. To begin with, even traversing the smooth London streets these vehicles jolt you to bits, whilst inside the smell of burnt gasoline is often stifling, so just imagine these unwieldy things bumping along over cobble stones and the loose sandy ruts of rough tracks among the sand-dunes, which constantly necessitated every one who could, dismounting and pushing behind and pulling by ropes in front, to get the vehicle into an upright position again, out of the ruts. When you have the picture of this before you, just think of the passengers---not healthy people on a penny bus ride, but wounded soldiers and sailors. Upon the brow of many Death had set his seal. All those inside passengers were either wounded in the abdomen, shot through the lungs, or pierced through the skull, often with their brains running out through the wound, whilst we had more than one case of men with broken backs. Many of these had just been operated upon.

We started from the Boulevard Leopold at 3 in the afternoon. We arrived in Ghent at 5.30 next morning. For twenty-four hours those men had had no nourishment, and we were so placed that it was impossible to reach them. Now that you understand the circumstances, I will ask you to accompany me on that journey.

Leaving our own shell-swept street which seemed like hell let loose, we turned down a long boulevard. From one end to the other the houses were a sheet of flames. We literally travelled through a valley with walls of fire. Keeping well in the middle of the street we constantly had to make detours to avoid large shell-holes. At last we arrived at one of the large squares near the Cathedral. That appeared to be intact, whilst the Belgians had taken Rubens' and Van Dyck's famous pictures and hidden them in the crypts.

Every sort of vehicle in existence filled that square. It would have been possible to have walked across on the top of the cars. The only way to get out of Antwerp was across the Scheldt by a pontoon-bridge made of barges with planks between. It would not bear too much traffic, so the authorities let the people and vehicles cross one by one, still looking at passports.

For one and a half hours we stood there waiting for our turn to come. Just after we were safely over a shell struck the bridge and broke it in half.

From Antwerp to St. Nicolas is about twenty miles. It was the Highway of Sorrow. Some people escaped in carriages and carts, but by far the greater number plodded on foot. It was now 5 P. M. on an October evening; there was a fine drizzling rain; it was cold and soon it was dark. Along that road streamed thousands, panic-stricken, cold, hungry, weary, homeless. Where were they going? Where would they spend the night? Here was a mother carrying her baby, around her skirts clung four of five children, small sisters of five or six carried baby-brothers of two years old. There was a donkey cart piled high with mattresses and bundles and swarming on it were bedridden old men and women and babies. Here was a little girl wheeling an old fashioned cot-perambulator, with an old grey-bearded man in it, his legs dangling over the edge. Suddenly a girl's voice called out of the darkness, "Oh Mees, Mees, take me and my leetle dog with you. I have lost my father and he has our money." So we gave her a seat on the spiral stairs outside.

Very soon all the ills that could happen to sick men came upon us. The jolting and agony made them violently sick. Seizing any utensil which had been saved from the theatre I gave it to them, and we kept that mademoiselle busy outside. All along the road we saw little groups, weary mothers sitting on the muddy banks of a ditch sharing the last loaf among the family. After some time of slow travelling we came to St. Nicolas. Here the peasants ran out warning us, "The Germans have taken the main road to Ghent and blown up the bridge." So we went on by little lanes and by-ways across the sanddunes and flat country that lie between Belgium and Holland.

We were very fortunate in having with us a Captain of the Belgian Boy Scouts. He knew the way and guided us. Soon the order went forth from car to car, "Lights out and silence!" Later on we saw the reason for this; across some sloping fields by a river we saw the tents and glimmering lights of the Germans. We passed very few houses, as we avoided towns and villages; any habitations we saw were shuttered and barred, for the people hid in terror expecting every one who passed to be the dreaded enemy. All this time our men were in torture, constantly they asked "Are we nearly there, Sister? How much longer?" I, who was strong, felt dead beat, so what must they have felt? One weary soul gave up the battle and just died. We could not even reach him to cover his face as he lay there among his companions.

From St. Nicolas I was faced with new anxiety. Where were our friends who went to Ghent with the first convoy of wounded? Had they taken the main road and fallen into the hands of the Germans? I thought of all the tales 1 had heard of the treatment Englishwomen received at their hands. At any place where people were visible we anxiously inquired if three buses had passed that way earlier. We could get no satisfactory answer.

Soon we began to meet the first detachments of the Expeditionary Force. In a narrow lane with a ditch on one side lay an overturned cannon whilst a plump English Major cursed and swore in the darkness. Then a heavy motor lorry confronted us; one of us had to back till a suitable place came in the narrow lane where we could pass. Later on we met small companies of weary Tommies, wet and footsore, who had lost their way. Our Scout Captain warned them to turn back, telling them the Germans had by now entered Antwerp, but they did not believe us. Even had they believed us, they had their orders to relieve Antwerp, so to Antwerp they went, never to return.

At last that weary night came to an end. For some hours I had been relieved by another nurse, and sat on top in the rain and cold. The medical students were so worn out that they lay down in the narrow passage between the seats and slept, oblivious of our trampling over them. Before dawn we entered the suburbs of Ghent.

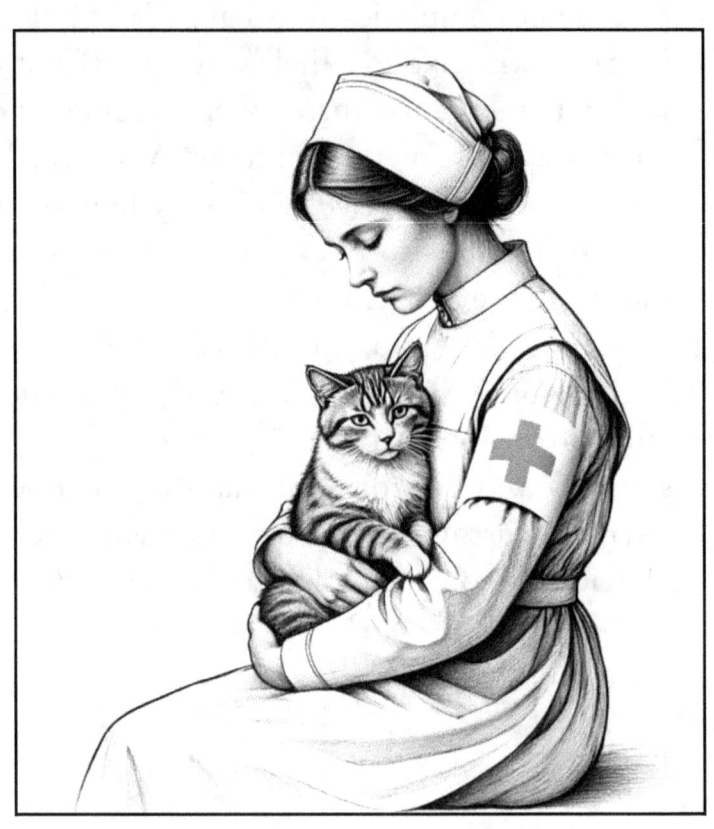

CHAPTER V
GHENT

WE drew up outside a railway station where a great hotel had been turned into a Red Cross Hospital. The young doctor, who had only just got to bed, received us without enthusiasm, telling us they were "full." This gentleman afterwards joined our party and was one of our most hard-working surgeons. He had heard nothing of other buses from Antwerp. Meanwhile, I stood out in the square and refused to be comforted, protesting that if they did not rise up and find them I would go no farther, but return and search those German tents for my friend. So one of the young doctors said that just as soon as we had disposed of the wounded in hospitals he would come and help me search.

The British wounded we all placed in one bus and brought with us to our journey's end, excepting one officer. He was so ill it would have killed him. So a young lady, a V. A. D. nurse, stayed with him in a Catholic Hospital, but the Germans let her go later on, when he was well.

We placed a few patients in each hospital wherever they could find room, whilst we anxiously inquired if they had received our first convoy of patients, but we received no news. This done, our Chief told us all to meet at 9 A. M. at a certain hotel for breakfast, after which we were to continue our journey to Bruges, as the Germans were marching forward. Then one of the doctors came with me on our search for the two missing ladies.

At the station we hired an old basket-carriage; the driver taking us for a party of trippers come to see the sights! I had secured the names of fourteen leading hotels, but either my French was so bad or his head so dull that he took us to see the Botanical Gardens! On our journey we went through the poor localities.

Down a little street I suddenly spied a familiar war-grey motor car with a big Red Cross on the back. "Why, there is Mrs. W-----'s motor car!" I cried. We concluded the chauffeur had put up there for the night, for over a door was a lamp proclaiming "Night-Watchman." Imagine my surprise at finding both Mrs. W------ and my friend, G------, cosily tucked up in a four-poster bed, and quite amused at our anxiety! They had arrived at nine the night before.

After a hearty breakfast, the first meal we had

taken since 7.30 Wednesday evening (and this was Friday morning), we all mounted a motor-bus and had a pleasant, sunny ride to Bruges, with the promise of the week-end in that quaint little town to recuperate.

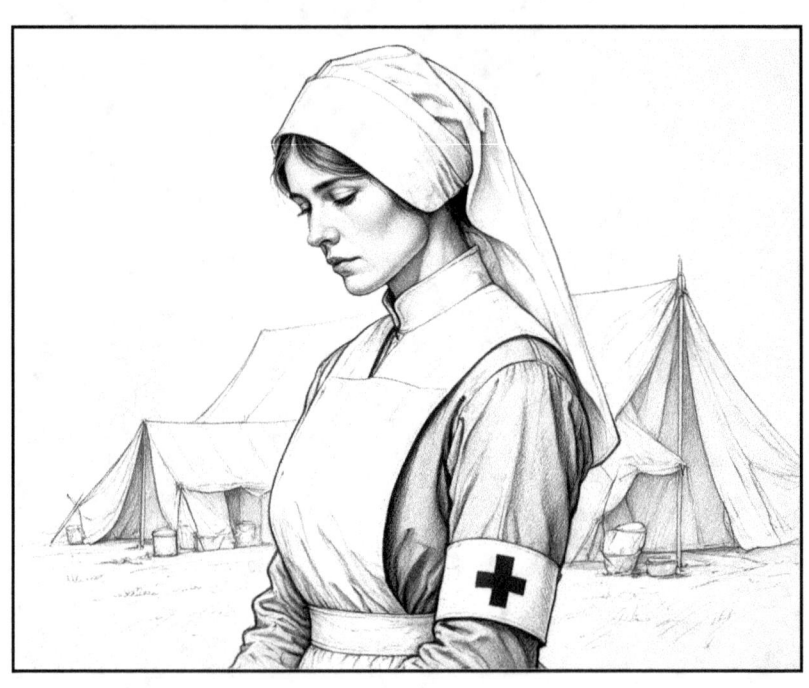

CHAPTER VI
BRUGES

ARRIVING at Bruges we found the usually quiet little town alive with bustle and excitement. The market place was astir with warlike activities; cavalry, artillery and lorries filled the square; smart young officers, keen and alert, gave orders; horses were being groomed; all was hopefulness and keen expectation. The hotels were full, so we were quartered, two or three in different pensions. Ours was down a winding network of alley-ways, over a canal. This Division was part of the British Expeditionary Force. They were just off to the Relief of Antwerp. We watched them march away, so assured of victory. It is hard to think that those splendid men, the number of them running well into five figures, never came back. Either prisoners in Germany or going over the borderland into Holland, they were interned in weary captivity. But that sunny morning there was no room for foreboding shadows. We nurses were usually kept in ignorance of the why and wherefore of our movements, and to us, with our inability to grasp the general situation, it seemed as though we spent our time flying in unnecessary haste. With all this great force of British soldiers gone to relieve Antwerp, added to those already there, why fear? I overheard one of our men say, "I wish we had all these women safe in England," and the conclusion we came to was, they all funked having a lot of women in their charge and foresaw troubles that would never come.

That afternoon a party of our people went over to Ostend to see what arrangements could be made for a hospital there; we were included in the joyride. Once there, my friend and I held a consultation. To put it shortly, it resulted in this. We had come to Belgium to nurse the Belgians; what society we served under was a matter of indifference to us. If our party chose to go home to England, we meant to stay. Why all this haste in flying from town to town? (As subsequent events proved, our flight had been quite necessary.) So we quietly went round to the Belgian Croix Rouge and offered our services. They accepted us with open arms, for patients were many and nurses few. They offered us La Plage Hotel with 657 bedrooms! We explained that we would come back early the following week, and then returned with our party to Bruges.

On the way our car broke down near Zeebrugge,

and some jolly Tommies lifted us into their motor lorry; it was great fun! When we returned we found the lady-farmers and another lady, a General's wife. We took them into our confidence, and asked them if they would like to help at La Plage Hotel. They were enthusiastic, for we saw no prospect of work in the near future until another hospital equipment had been procured. We then went home to our different pensions.

At 2 A. m. one of the doctors came running round, saying the Germans were marching on Bruges, that we must fly at once to the market-place and that all must start within half an hour for Ostend. We quickly dressed, lugging our heavy holdalls down confusing back streets, scattering shoes and brushes in our wake. Two of the medical students could not be found, as we did not know their address. To our disgust we went off without them. This all confirmed our previous impression (a false impression) of unnecessary flight. We were glad that we had work to do elsewhere. On our journey we found a broken down car, and were asked to help. Who should the driver be but Philip Gibbs, the famous war correspondent. We came into Ostend together, and later on, we saw a good deal of him, as he often shared our meals at Furnes.

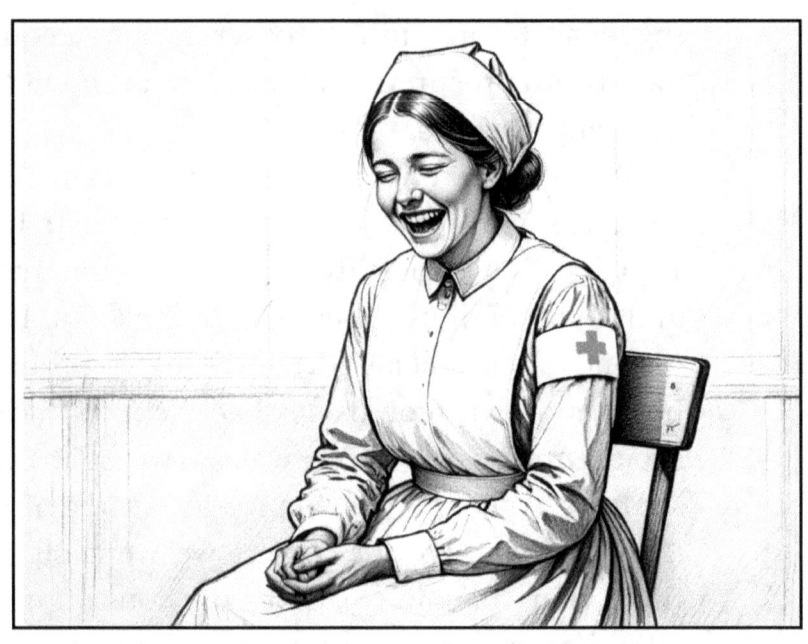

CHAPTER VII
OSTEND

IT was 4 A. M. when we arrived at Ostend, dark, cold and wet. All the hotels were overflowing because all Belgium had converged on Ostend. We came to the Casino, a huge showy building which had been turned into a British Red Cross Hospital. In one large hall were five hundred beds filled with wounded. The Sisters were kind; here and there was an empty bed, so they said we might lie down on these among the patients till six o'clock, when we must turn out for them to wash the men. The time came all too soon; we were aroused and turned out on to the wet street. We then found our Chief and told him we had joined the Belgian Croix Rouge. Proceeding to the Central office, we were followed closely by the fox terrier whom I had christened "Bombe."

They gave us six boy scouts to run our errands, a motor ambulance, and placed two doctors over the hospital. The doctors were father and son; the elder man a noted eye-specialist. Arrived at the palatial hotel we found we were in charge of the whole of it with the exception of the right wing, which was occupied by the Russian Ambassador and his suite. The dining hall had been emptied of furniture and mattrasses had been placed on the floor, the authorities not wishing the beautiful bedroom furniture to be used. A cook was also provided. Besides there were the four lady-farmers and Mrs. C-----, all most devoted workers.

Very soon the patients arrived, seventy of them, not seriously wounded. They consisted chiefly of pneumonias, typhoids and wounded convalescents. On the whole we thoroughly enjoyed that week-end in Ostend. We spent Sunday, Monday and Tues day there, feeling the work a great responsibility, and busy catering for and nursing our large family without a moment's rest. Some of our party dropped in and looked round; and we really felt we had taken a wise step, for they had no work, and were sleeping where they could, whilst the weather was atrocious.

The entrance hall of La Plage Hotel is a thing of costly splendour, the roof a big dome inlaid with mosaics. At night our cook went home, likewise the boy scouts. There was no one left to guard all this magnificence, and we two felt hugely responsible, so we sent our lady-helpers upstairs to bed whilst we dragged one of the patient's mattrasses to the front door. Placing it on the floor as a barrier we slept there. This served two purposes, we were near the patients and could also answer the door quickly.

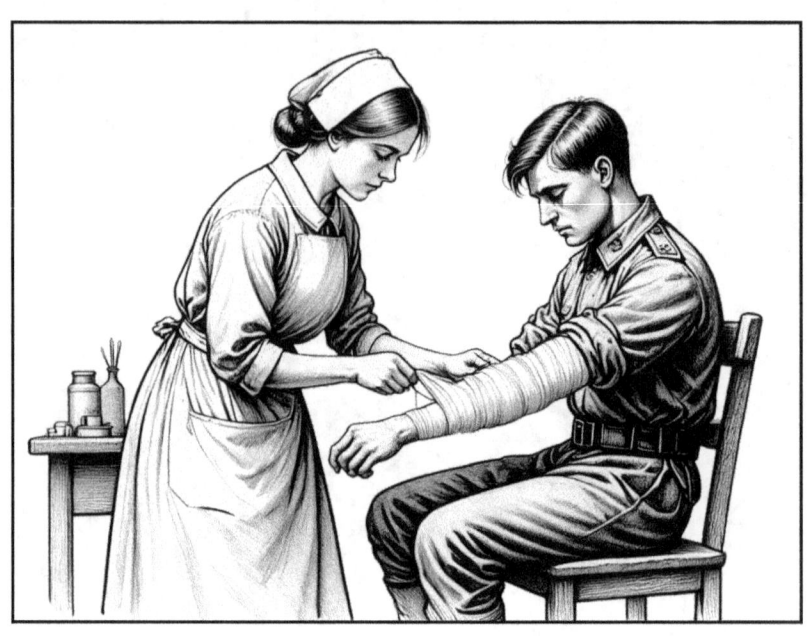

CHAPTER VIII
THE EVACUATION

TUESDAY night was a night of alarms; there was one interruption after another. First a drunken man walked in, announcing that he belonged to the nobility, that his mother was the head of all the Croix Rouge, and he wanted a shirt. We could not find a shirt, but we had a chest protector; that pleased him mightily! Finding the place warm he refused to go away, so we bolted up the stairs and locked ourselves in one of the bedrooms. After some time we ventured forth to find he had gone. We settled down again on our mattrass with the faithful Bombe at our feet. Then an officer came in at 11 P. M. and ordered all our soldiers to be down at the great terminus-station (the station we first arrived at) by 12 midnight. We found their clothes and dressed them.

Fortunately I had laid in seventy brown loaves, having heard that there might be a scarcity; the coffee was also over the fire, ready for breakfast. We gave them each a mugful. and a loaf. It was very sad to see those poor fellows limp and hobble out in a large body. The station was nearly a mile away; it was wet and dark and they were unfit to walk. Those who could support the others, gave a willing shoulder or arm, and so they left us, leaning on each other---halt, lame and blind.

Earlier in the evening one of our doctors came round and told us that our party were leaving for England the following day, as the Germans were not far away. He told us that Ostend meant to make a big fight; the British Navy would fire over the city upon the besieging Germans, and it was not safe for civilians to stay. But we had thrown in our lot with the Belgians and meant to stick to them, so we declined to leave.

After the patients had departed we replaced our mattrass and went to sleep. Suddenly we were rudely awakened by the door bursting open and a tall Garde Civique shouted out in French, "Everybody is to arise and fly!" We went upstairs to call our friends; by mistake I opened the wrong door, the door of an apparently empty room. To my surprise I found a strange woman in bed. This led to a general discovery. The building was filled with strangers, people who had slunk in by some back door unknown to us. I taught my friend the French for the warning sentence of the Garde Civique, and we each took alternate floors of this immense building, opening each door and shouting "Everybody is to arise and fly!" It was quite amusing to see the queer assortment of refugees that popped their heads out of those doors and gathered in the corridors; bald-headed old men in pyjamas, fat, flurried old women and girls. During the next hour we watched these figures slinking down the stairs and hurrying away like rats forsaking a sinking ship. Also the Russian Ambassador and his suite, wrapped in fur coats, drove away in their white automobile, and we were left alone. We again packed up our holdalls, removed them to the front door and sat on them.

Very soon Dr. Van O----- and his son came round. They urged us to accept our chance to escape to England. The white-haired old man spoke with great pathos; he said that he and his son were Ostend citizens. They would share the city's fate for good or ill, and help their fellow-countrymen. But for English women to remain at the mercy of the German hordes was rash imprudence. Just then the young doctor came back, saying they were soon to sail, and urging us to join them. He said that an ambulance would fetch us at 6 A. M., and that a lady of great influence and wealth, who was interested in our hospital, had procured for us a means of transport.

Three of the Harwich to Antwerp steamers were

secured to take over the wounded to England.

Each ship was equipped for five hundred wounded, even orderlies had been provided. Eleven o'clock had come, but still no sign of an ambulance; I went round to the quay and found our party. They had not forgotten us, but an unfortunate accident had happened in the midst of all that traffic and turmoil.

A chauffeur had set out with a beautiful new Red Gross car; the traffic was appalling. As you know, on the Continent vehicles drive to the right. This Englishman had always driven to the left. A crisis occurred in the rush of vehicles. Following the habit of a lifetime, he moved to the left, collided with another vehicle, and tipped over into the canal. He escaped unhurt but there was no time to save the, car. All this muddle nearly caused us to be left behind. I hastened back, hailing a passing ambulance, and literally commandeering the unwilling driver by threats and entreaties to take us to the quay.

Finally we arrived just before the boat started. My little dog, Bombe, was hidden under my violet cloak, but just as we were crossing the draw-bridge, a passport officer spied him as he popped his head out at an unfortunate moment, "No dogs allowed, Miss; must be put in quarantine forty days;" so I had to abandon him. On the quay stood Miss

B-----, the rich lady who had procured the steamers for us. To me she was a stranger, but, seeing my distress, she smilingly said she would find a home for him.

The quay was a scene of heart-rending sights. It was crowded with panic-stricken refugees. They knelt down, imploring us to take them. Just as the steamer loosed her moorings some sprang over the edge, hanging on to the ship's railing; we pulled them into safety. Others fell into the water and were drowned.

Down below in the saloon the stretchers were laid side by side. Amongst the hundreds of sufferers we recognized many of the men we had nursed in Antwerp, and were hailed joyfully. De Rasquinet had been left behind in Ghent, but, to my delight, there was the little man whom I had tried to save when the first convoy started from Antwerp. A few days later we met him again in the London Hospital, when visiting the wards set aside for the Belgian wounded.

Ambulance trains, with military sisters and doctors in charge, met the steamers at Dover. In a businesslike and methodical manner they took over our boys---the men whose sufferings we had shared, with whom we had passed through the horrors of war. It was splendid to have them well provided for, but we hated parting from them.

Next morning we all went up to London, a sad, travel-worn little party. We had nothing left, no hospital equipment, no prospect of more work, and life seemed flat after the stirring events through which we had just passed. We lunched together at Charing Cross Hotel; our Chief took all our addresses in case there might be another hospital started in the future, but just then it was "goodbye." Meanwhile, returning to our friends, we found ourselves the heroines of the hour. Having no other clothes, we sailed around London in our violet cloaks, white military caps and conspicuous red crosses, swinging German helmets on our arms! After three days we returned to my friend's home in the same town as our old hospital, there to receive an enthusiastic welcome.

PART II

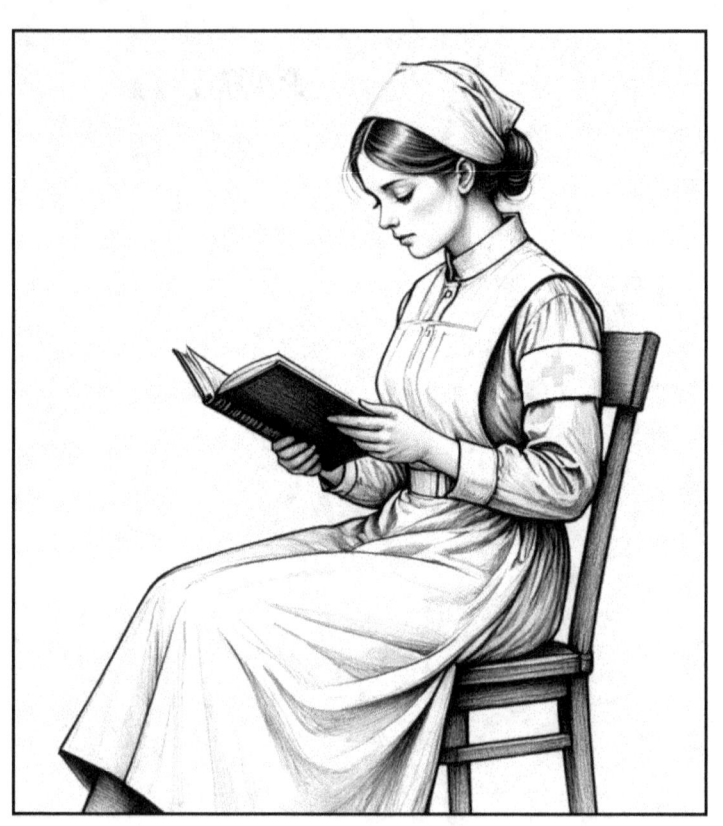

CHAPTER IX
FURNES

ON October 18th, just five days after the dispersal of our hospital at Charing Cross, a telegram was handed to us, saying "Meet the nine-thirty boat train, Victoria, tonight." In delighted excitement we again packed our holdalls and caught the train to London. At Victoria we were met by our kind friend, Mr. Souttar, the eminent London Hospital surgeon. We found that our hospital staff had left the previous night, and owed our being included in it to Mr. Souttar. Either we were difficult to reach in a hurry, or they had not forgotten our independence at Ostend, but we certainly should have been overlooked had it not been for this gentleman. We were placed in charge of the Duchess of Sutherland, who had a hospital unit at St. Malo, a suburb of Dunkerque. Arrived there we spent the next day and night at the St. Malo Hotel. The Germans gave us a warm reception that night; a squadron of airplanes bombarded Dunkerque, shelling the quays where the ammunition was stored. We leaned out of window, gazing over the sea at the battle in the air, listening the while to loud explosions.

Our new hospital was located in Furnes, a quaint little town fifteen miles to the east of Dunkerque, and about three or four miles west of Nieuport, whilst the seaside resort of La Panne was just two or three miles to the north. Ypres was fifteen to twenty miles south of Furnes. Each day an ambulance drove into Dunkerque for the mail and to buy provisions. It was this ambulance that took us out to our new sphere of work.

The building in which we worked was a large Roman Catholic College; the principal and professors were still living in it. It was a large rambling building covering a good deal of ground. There were two big courtyards, one of them devoted to the motor-cars and ambulances, which really formed a squadron. Across the inner courtyard from the main part was a building containing two large classrooms on the ground floor, and upstairs one huge dormitory where we all slept. There were other small class-rooms round, which served several purposes: laundry, wards and operation-theatre.

The scene in that great place was one of bustling life and activity all the twenty-four hours round. In spite of constant contact with suffering, misery and death, to us doctors and nurses there was a great share of happiness and the joy of life. It is a great thing to feel you are fighting death and saving heroes, besides which we were a very happy crowd. There were now twenty-six nurses, mostly new ones; we had with us the same three medical students and two or three of our former men-doctors, but the four lady-doctors had left us, and in their place we had three or four new men-doctors and one lady-doctor as an anæsthetist and surgical store-keeper.

The lady-farmers had left us, and the number of non-medical people was reduced to a minimum. Now, for the first time, we had orderlies---the ex-professors became our willing helpers and the most devoted and capable attendants of the patients. I cannot speak highly enough of them. These men, who had spent their lives as leaders of classes, cleaned grates, swept floors, scrubbed and attended to all the menial wants of the patients. By degrees the younger amongst them were taken by the army and replaced by men released from Holland who, under the Treaty of Geneva, must not fight again.

At that time Furnes was the Headquarters of the Belgian Army, and the quaint Hôtel de Ville, dating from 1582, was King Albert's Army Quarters. The old-world market square was filled with every sort of war vehicle; officers occupied the inns and soldiers swarmed everywhere, sleeping at night in the Cathedral and another great church where straw was spread on the floor for them. Queen Elizabeth lived at La Panne, where there were hospitals and many convalescents. It was never shelled.

We lived in Furnes from October 18th to January 15th. All the time we were in Belgium we were never out of hearing of the constant boom and thunder of artillery, and at night the sky was afire with the battle going on to the east of us, about three miles away. Our life was a complex thing to describe; there was a constant coming and going of outsiders. People came to Furnes to see things---great people. The college being large and other accommodation in the town nil, we put them up, and they were our guests for the time being.

Attached to us was a most interesting body of people, "The Munro Ambulance Corps." Dr. Munro was its chief. He is now Sir Hector Munro. With him, driving ambulances, were many well. known people; just a few names I remember---Lady Dorothy Feilding, the eldest son of General Melisse, head of the Belgian R. A. M. C., Dr. Jellett, the Dublin gynæcologist; Claude and Alice Askew, the novelists (since drowned in a submarine attack); Miss McNaughton, authoress; Mrs. Knocker and Miss Chisholme; Mr. Hunt of Yokohama and Mr.

Sekkar, a great sport and our good friend. All their ambulances were stored in our front yard, numbering over twenty. With them were four jolly young gentlemen-amateur chauffeurs who soon became our friends. These people worked mostly at night, gathering the wounded and removing them under cover of darkness. We received all those who could not travel further into France.

Our dining-room was great! It was really the kitchen. A big stove covered with immense pots occupied one side. In front of it stood our chef, an ex-patient named Maurice. He was the sunniest fellow I ever met. He came in with the first batch of Furnes wounded, shot through the throat. When he laughed it sounded like a tin whistle blown by an amateur. He had been a cook, and when he was well the Queen gave him to us as chef. He wore a baker's cap and apron, presiding at all the festivities. Under him were seven refugee nuns in voluminous black dresses and white caps like airplanes. They peeled potatoes and washed dishes. There were three trestle-tables covered with check oilcloth; we each helped ourselves to an enamel pint-mug, lead spoon and fork, and taking a bowl to the stove it was filled with coffee, soup or "bullybeef."

For several weeks we lived on that stand-by of our Tommies. Disguise it as you will, in pie, rissole or curry, hide it under all the Parisian names you can find in a French cookery-book, at the first taste it just jumps up and shouts "Here we are again!" The other three articles which comprised our menu were coarse, wet, black bread, rancid butter from the Tommies' rations, and a dainty which resembled a bath-room-tile in size, shape and consistency, and which I firmly believe was Spratt's Dog Biscuits!

We all sat together at these crowded tables, lords and ladies, chauffeurs, doctors and nurses. Once even, later on, we gave a dinner party, our guest being no less a personage than a Royal Prince of England. After the sun set the most impressive feature in Furnes was the darkness. Every house was shrouded in gloom. The streets were black. Our hospital was invisible except for a glimmering candle or cheap, evil-smelling lamp here and there. Never shall I forget that first night! The Battle of the Yser had just begun, and before we had got settled we were inundated with stretchers laden with groaning, bleeding men. By a guttering candle we examined their wounds.

My friend and I, with two new Sisters, were in charge of a large ward, one of the big class-rooms. We were awfully short of all the appliances we consider indispensable to a hospital. Many of our beds consisted of sacking filled with straw or shavings. We rarely had a sheet and no mackintoshes in those early days. Stretchers lay all over the floor with men who were covered with mud and blood. In our ward there was a little elderly lady who quietly offered her services, and as she looked capable I sent her to clear away the evening meal and wipe down the tables. She never bothered me again but quietly busied herself setting things in order.

Soon two big oil-lamps relieved the darkness and some large scissors that we had longed for lay to hand to rip the men's clothes off them. The unassuming little helper had been out to buy them. A few days after, when we had time to breathe, we were introduced. It was Miss McNaughton, the writer of "A Lame Dog's Diary" and other books.

She stayed with us several days helping in our ward. After that she procured a tiny room at the station and ran a soup-kitchen for the wounded. Now, this sounds a homely and commonplace sort of occupation, but when you realize the circumstances you will know what courage it required.

As I said before, Furnes was the Army Headquarters. King Albert spent most of his time there, and it was filled with military. Also Furnes station was the junction for all the little local railways that ran out to villages and towns at the Front, now so well known to all of us. One constantly heard the guard shouting "Poelcappelle!"

"Nieuport!" "Dixmude!" and many other names mentioned constantly in our present offensive. All the fresh troops and ammunition passed through here; all the wounded returned through here at night. Therefore Furnes, with the station as the bullseye of the target, was the constant centre of attention of the German artillery and airplanes.

Miss McNaughton was in the thick of it. She was a delicate little woman, highly strung and nervous, therefore it was particularly courageous of her to spend most of her time there peeling vegetables and stoking up furnaces. Often during that late autumn and winter when we had finished work we would take an after-supper walk to her tiny kitchen, a merry party of us. Sitting on sacks of potatoes and onions we would give her a hand preparing the midnight soup. Then, when the long ambulance trains shunted in at twelve, we would sally forth with trays of steaming mugs filled with hot soup and coffee, and, boarding the trains, give the eager sufferers on the stretchers a good hot drink to warm them up. Several shells hit the station. Once, when the collector was clipping tickets, his clipper was knocked out of his hand and his thumb blown off, whilst a thick pocket book over his heart saved his life, a piece of shrapnel being embedded in it.

After Christmas, Miss McNaughton moved to La Panne. That was when Furnes had grown too unhealthy for human beings. We spent a happy Sunday with her at her villa, where she was writing a book about her experiences. A young clergyman, who was one of our chauffeurs, went over to take a service at La Panne Hospital, so, as we three were all Miss McNaughton's friends, he took us along. We had quite an exciting time, coming home along the Ypres-Furnes Road. A Taube, spotting the Red Cross on top, thought he had some wounded to kill, so he followed us for miles, dropping shrapnel. It was great fun! I looked longingly at the fragments falling all over the road, but could not prevail on the parson to pull up whilst we gathered a few bits for presents to our home people. That clergyman was a great sport. He was not like a parson at all. Not only was he a chauffeur, but he was a Boy Scout troop commander and a skilled engineer and carpenter. We nurses were constantly indebted to him for shelves, stools, cosy corners, and other useful ward-furniture made out of old sugar cases, etc., in his spare time. The following spring while he was waiting for a batch of wounded at a dressing station, he used to go out into the fields and pick us nosegays of cowslips till bullets whistling through his hair made him realize that "discretion was the better part of valour." That young man afterwards went with General Townsend to the Relief of Kut, and was promoted a Captain. The Turks sent a bullet through his head, but after a few months' convalescence in India he is back at his post again, "Somewhere."

The reader must excuse all these excursions on to side-tracks. The fact is, nothing in our life was consecutive at Furnes, or later at Hoogestadt. It was just a series of pictures made up of interesting events and people.

First of all, at Furnes, there was a mad rush of work. While the Battle of the Yser was proceeding every nerve was strained day and night to cope with the work. Then after two or three weeks things died down to a few casualties each day. During that time we assumed more the nature of a Base-Hospital, and instead of packing off all who could travel next morning in ambulances, we nursed them to something approaching convalescence, or till another rush came. We had permanently attached to us two Belgian Colonels, a Major and some Lieutenants who examined the wounded each morning, placing tickets over the beds of those who were to be moved to France and England.

All this time the roar of heavy artillery went on by day and night. After dark we could trace the battle-line all along the east, from north to south by the blaze of guns and flares. Often Belgian and French airplanes would engage in sharp contests right over our heads, as the Taubes dropped their bombs down on the streets below. We all ran out to watch who would win, and once I saw a Taube hit, and fire burst out of its tail as it volplaned towards the cast in a cloud of smoke. Very soon after these little affairs some stretchers would arrive with wounded civilians.

We had been in Furnes about ten days, when, late one evening, a proclamation was issued that we were to retire immediately to Poperinghe, so we all packed into the ambulances and sped away. No one gave us any reason; to us it was a joy-ride, but I suppose the authorities thought the Germans were about to break the line and enter Furnes. We went at a breakneck speed along dark country lanes, and at places the roads reminded one of an Arabian Night's Tale. By a little copse were pitched some tents, fires were burning on the ground, and attached to tripods pots were boiling, while Arab-Sheiks with white flowing garments, gay turbans, scarves and swarthy beards squatted around or at. tended to their horses.

At Poperinghe we found the British, and squares and streets were bustling with military life. The French were there also. How grand were the French Cuirassiers, seated on their handsome horses, wearing shining brass helmets and breastplates, while from the back of the helmets swept red or black plumes!

As usual, all the inns were filled with military. We came to a little estaminet where we all crowded in for a meal in the bar-room. But there was no sleeping accommodation. About midnight the nurses were quartered in a convent the other side of the town but we lost our way, and finally, tired out, found ourselves in the little white beds, enclosed with curtains, of a huge dormitory.

We spent three days at Poperinghe, when we were all taken back to Furnes again. Evidently the Germans found it too tough a job to break through. For the next two months we nursed French soldiers, as French troops were fighting on that section of the Front. It becomes almost monotonous to tell you again that all those hundreds and hundreds of men we nursed were far spent---suffering from shock collapse, excessive hemorrhage, broken to pieces, many mortally wounded, all in agony, suffering from cold, hunger, exposure to winter weather, frost bite, and every evil that can bring strong men to death's door. We had also a new trouble to contend with, gangrene had broken out, often of a malignant description. We isolated these and amputated limbs where possible to save them.

Tetanus appeared, but we soon obtained serums from England and gave all patients with wounds covering large surfaces a preventive injection. Often large pieces of clothing were embedded in wounds, to say nothing of shrapnel and mud. From beneath one man's shoulder-blade we even extracted a large brass time-fuse! We had one wonderful case of recovery in our large ward; an officer, with the rank of Major, was brought in with huge wounds in his abdomen, while his intestines were absolutely riddled with shot. The surgeons cut out twelve feet of entrails, and he made an excellent recovery! This was the more remarkable considering that all the patients surrounding him were suffering from dirty and festering wounds, and at that time we had no means of sterilizing the ward dressings. Later on we had large steam sterilizers in the theatre.

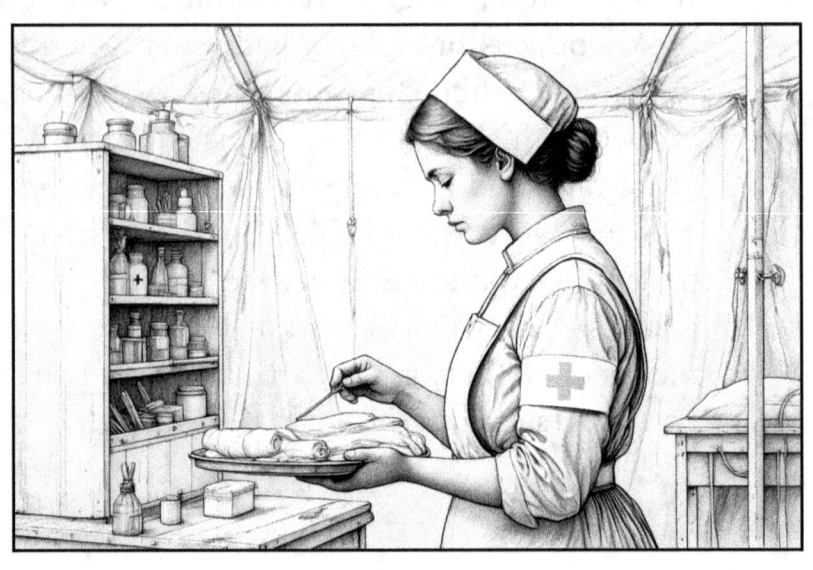

CHAPTER X
FIRING THE "SOIXANTE-QUINZE"'

I TOLD you that in Furnes we nursed the French. That remark needs qualifying. Not only did we nurse the French "poilu," but amongst them were representatives from all the French colonies, black, brown and yellow men. Great black, woolly-haired Senegalese from East Africa, savages and cannibals, lay stretched out on our beds, or oftener on the floors, for we were overflowing. These poor fellows could not even speak French, and they suffered bitterly from the cold. As we passed them they would hold up big bandaged hands, wailing "Oh! Madame, oh! la! la! la! la!" There were also Turcos with red fezzes and baggy trousers, Zouaves with cutaway jackets, Algerians and Arab-Spahis with peculiar bowl-shaped turbans. Among them were Annamites from the Orient, members of the Legion-Étrangers, and French Alpinos with blue tam-o'-shanters.

One night we received Mr. R-----, editor of a

noted sporting-paper. He had been out on a Munro ambulance and had run into a German scout party. The ambulance made a spurt for liberty. Mr. R----- sprang to the back of the car and hung on, at the same time being shot through both legs, which were broken. He was dragged along the road whilst the car bolted for life, the Germans firing after them. Even with both legs badly broken, he could not refrain from joking. We had him removed to England as soon as possible.

Mr. Sekkar, one of the Munro chauffeurs, was just loading up a car, when a piece of shrapnel made a great wound in his leg. He did not mention it, but continued to drive the car to Furnes whilst the blood ran on to the foot-board. He received no attention until he got to Furnes.

There was a certain little station just near the trenches which the Munro party often visited. Gathering the wounded from a dressing-station by the trenches, they drove them to the ambulance-trains waiting at this station. One November day I was taken out on one of the cars. We came to a place where four roads met, and here our ambulances pulled up. Just by the cross-ways was a battery of three French 75's. I sat on the car and watched them firing for a while, then, getting used to the deafening roar and trembling earth, I gradually drew nearer. On the ground were shells which looked like giant thermos-flasks, some red and some khaki; one colour burst up in the air as a timed, explosion; others burst upon contact.

Mr. Sekkar had said "Don't go too near, or you will be deaf." So I kept a little way off, near the officer who was shouting orders. It was most engrossing watching the great oven-door at the back open with clock work precision and the two soldiers lift in the shell and bolt the locks. Then, walking round to the side of the wheels, a soldier took a cord, gave it a sharp jerk, and lo!---the whole earth rocked. Flames shot out in a circle all round the rear of the gun, and the air was rent with an appalling roar. Then you heard the shell on its journey of eight or twelve miles, roaring, buzzing and humming off into the distance, followed by a faraway explosion.

One cannon after another performed this feat, with two minutes pause between each. Then there was some shifting of the gun into position again. The Major looked down at me and said, "Would you like to have a shot at the Boches?" and I said "Rather!" "All right. Put some wool in your ears, take hold of that string when I give the word and pull smartly!" I have often wondered where that shell landed and with what result.

Returning to my seat in the car we watched the German shells ploughing up the fields all round.

What hundreds of shells they wasted trying to hit that battery!

Everywhere in the fields in front of us the earth went up in dense clouds, leaving hills and holes behind. The little paved avenue in front of us was a "hot" place. It was impossible for us to traverse it till they moved their range to another spot. The Boches never got that battery, though they nearly got us. After dark they gave up the job, so we proceeded about half a mile down the lane, where we came to a dilapidated cottage. Out of the darkness we saw staggering soldiers, leaning on each other, flounder into the straw-strewn room.

Stretchers arrived constantly, borne by Red-Cross orderlies. We were used to death and dying at our hospital, but here we met despair. Most of those lying on that straw were in extremis---nothing could be done for them, grey ashen faces looked dully at us, they were mostly too bad to groan. It is dreadful to be impotent, to stand by grievously stricken men it is impossible to help, to see the death-sweat gathering on young faces, to have no means of easing their last moments. This is the nearest to Hell I have yet been. We put all the hopeful cases into our cars, driving one or two loads to the little station, and then returning for more, which we took back with us to Furnes.

Towards the end of November we took over the

operation-theatre. Things were quieter then, as the Flemish mud made an offensive impossible. There was only the usual artillery-fire and small raids to deal with. Meanwhile a very cold winter had commenced. It was pitiful to see those poor Belgian soldiers without any comfortable quarters when out of the trenches. My friend and I had hired a bed-room in the town. We were very lucky, for our landlady was goodness itself to us. Just opposite our house there was a church built on the generous lines of a cathedral, and here a large detachment of soldiers was quartered, sleeping on straw on the stone flags. We used to watch them at dawn come out in the deep snow to a horse-trough, and, breaking the ice, strip to their waists and wash. After dusk we saw them marching in from the trenches in their ragged blue overcoats, caked in mud, carrying piles of accoutrement on their backs and spades and guns over their shoulders.

No warm home-coming for them, no fire to dry their clothes by, no hot meal ready. Just the dark, cold church. These men had no bundle of letters from home to cheer them; all they had to face was a desolated country, desecrated firesides, ruined homes, starving penniless families, violated womenfolk and suspense---not just for weeks or months, but for years, without news of all that life held dear for them. Do you wonder that they hate the Germans? In return they were paid three-halfpence per day. A few weeks ago I received a letter from a Belgian Captain whom I had nursed. He writes "Dear Sister, do you realize that it is now three years since I have received any news of my wife and three little ones? Are they alive or dead? The suspense has made an old man of me; at thirty-five my hair has turned grey with anxiety."

Most of our operations occurred at night, as the wounded travelled through the danger-zone with less risk of being fired upon after dark. During the day we performed operations on patients who had been in the wards for some time. Our doctors and nurses had no cosy sitting-room to rest in when off duty. There was only the busy kitchen stove for warmth; so we used to gather them in the theatre when there was no case to prepare for. What jolly times I remember in between the rushes of work! Our stove was always going, with a big kettle of boiling water ready for emergency cases, so about eleven A. M., after the nurses and doctors had done the morning round of dressings, we used to make a cup of tea.

One of the chauffeurs would bring in from Dunkerque a box of French pastries, or better still, some kind mother sent a lovely "tuck-box" containing an English homemade cake! Then the men would find their hair needed a barber's attention, so out came some scissors and a sheet, and we became pro tem. a hair-dresser's establishment! During the autumn rush of the Battle of the Yser we had so overflowed our borders that we were obliged to take in two small class-rooms, scattering straw thickly on the floor in lieu of mattrasses. It was a miserable arrangement, but better than the streets. Later on, in December, one of the class-rooms was turned into a sitting room for the staff. The couches consisted of crates, covered with red blankets; an old bedstead boarded up at one side, with a sack of shavings and blankets over it, made a fine Chesterfield couch! The students hired a gramophone and piano from Dunkerque, so we became quite civilized.

.

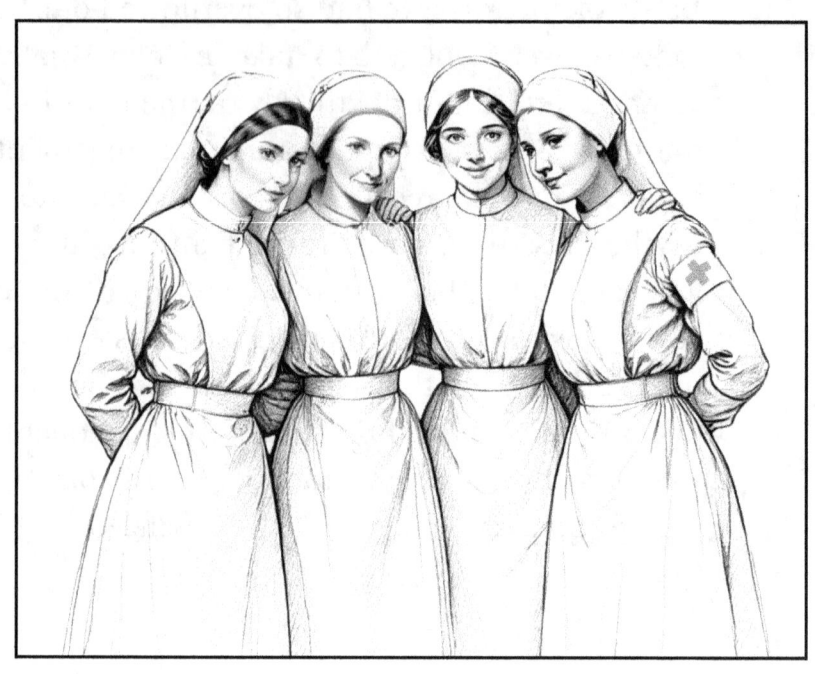

CHAPTER XI
CHRISTMAS

DECEMBER had arrived, and Christmas was approaching. We felt the excitement of it in the air. Every one wrote long letters home, asking for good things for all our hundred or more patients. The home-folk responded, and soon big crates arrived, both for patients and staff. My friend and I had a memorable joy-ride to Dunkerque. After months of darkness, mud and shuttered shops, what a delight to see gay streets filled with stores, all gorgeous in a Christmas fairyland of decoration.

Dunkerque is a wonderful city; one day all the shops are shut and barred, sand-bags block the cellar gratings and the city retires underground! The town is receiving the attention of a German airplane squadron or of some siege guns over twenty miles away. After blowing up a few houses and digging some shell-holes in the streets the enemy "lets up" and everything is quiet again. The people scramble like ants out of an ant-hill, and all the gay life begins again!

There was a certain bazaar at Dunkerque, a big departmental-store of cheap goods, which was a perfect fairyland of toys and Christmas presents. Now, my friend and I were deeply interested in a little orphanage near us at Furnes, where twenty war-orphans, boys from three to fifteen years old, were cared for by nuns. So we went to the bazaar and bought things that boys like, also presents for our friends. Then the doctor who drove us in, took us to a hotel dinner. All these seem ordinary events, but to us they were delightful excitements after having lived in a kitchen and eaten bully beef for months. We were like girls from boarding-school let out for a holiday!

We were by now doing night duty. We had a small ward of about twenty patients and the theatre. We two took the theatre or ward, for a week each, alternately. Every morning when fine we would go for long walks, either to La Panne or by the canals, sometimes accompanied by a doctor or the Munro chauffeurs. During December Furnes became colder and colder as regards temperature, thick snow lying everywhere. But as regards personal safety it grew hotter and hotter.

All the time we had stayed there Taubes and guns shelled us once or twice a week, but now it was a daily occurrence. From two to four o'clock every afternoon we were awakened by loud explosions. G----- would say to me in a sleepy voice, "Do you think that is the hospital gone?" It never occurred to us that a shell might dig a hole in our bed-room.

You know there are two classes of people in the world who have diametrically different views when in personal danger. One set are the right sort to go to the Front. The other kind should not live in Europe at present. They should go farming in Canada! They are best described by quoting a little story I saw in one of our comic papers lately. It ran something like this:---"Bill! What's a h'optimist and a pessimist?" (Bill) ---"Wall, I reckon as a h'optimist is one as thinks as them 'Uns is shooting of shells indiscriminate-like, not meant for no one in particular, whilst a pessimist, 'e thinks that every bloomin' shell is fired straight for 'isself, and 'e is the darn target!" The optimist was the only person who had a good time in Furnes!

So Christmas Eve arrived. We got no sleep that day. It was all hands to the wheel, nailing up festoons of gay bunting, holly, mistletoe and Christmas mottoes. Three big trees had to be procured and decorated with tinsel and hundreds of presents. Soldier stockings must be filled, so when they were asleep we night nurses tied one to each bed.

Never shall I forget the earlier hours of

Christmas morning! The partitions between two large class-rooms had been removed, making one very big ward of seventy or eighty patients. At one end of the ward an Altar had been fixed up with life-size plaster figures of the Virgin and Infant Christ; many tiny candles burning around. About 4.30 A. M. our little orphans, who were also choristers, filed in out of the darkness, robed in white; little acolytes in scarlet and lace waved chalices filled with smoking incense; priests in all the glory of the Romish vestments, with gold-embroidered stoles, stood before the Altar. Dim lights revealed the faces of the patients reverently lying in their beds. Such a motley crowd! Black Senegalese, Algerians, Frenchmen, Belgians, and here and there the cropped head of a German prisoner waiting for Absolution before the Altar that makes no distinction between friend and foe. Belgian orderlies stood with bowed heads at attention, and nurses continued to flit about noiselessly ministering to the helpless.

We were not present at the patient's Christmas Tree distribution, having gone to bed. But at three P.M. we rose and all the staff gathered in a hall of the Civilian Hospital across the way, where the orphans and staff had one tree between them. By four P. M. it was dark, and we were returning to our own hospital-grounds when shells began to fall---

Christmas cards from the Huns. The four night-nurses were free till eight P. M., when we took twelve hours' duty, so we were just having a game round the courtyard of hide-and-seek among the ambulances, the Munro chauffeurs chasing us with pieces of mistletoe. It seems a very incongruous pastime when a town is being bombarded!

Our Chief came to the door, ordering us in to take shelter. He had lately come from England and taken over the management, so was of course nervous of shells. But we had got so used to bombardments by now that it only added a little pleasurable excitement to an otherwise dull little town. My goodness, how those shells came down! Furnes had over two hundred shells in three quarters of an hour between four and five P. M. on Christmas Day. Afterwards the newspapers said there was an armistice and quite Christian good feeling between the two armies on Christmas Day!

All the Munro party dined with us that night. We had a real old-fashioned Christmas dinner. All the staff had received huge hampers of good things which were shared with the patients, who had a mid-day feast. We sat down to turkey, goose, sucking-pig, Christmas puddings all aflame, mince pies and dessert. Boxes of crackers were piled up and the old priest went down in his cellar and brought up some of his best wines. Soon every one was pulling crackers, reading idiotic mottoes, arrayed in ridiculous head-dresses, blowing tin whistles and every kind of "musical" toy. In the midst of all this revelry the great gate-bell clanged, and stretcher after stretcher arrived. Doctors hastily sprang from the table, still wearing clown's paper caps, and the half-eaten dinner lay forgotten, whilst the aftermath of the bombardment arrived in our theatre. So we passed from sunshine to storm, gathering honey where we might, and dropping the cup raised halfway to the lips when duty called.

That night, among our wounded soldiers, lay two little children and a young woman. A tot of two years old had both feet blown off; a little girl of four was minus an arm, and the woman had her leg blown off just below the hip and her arm broken. We had no separate ward to put them in, so put a screen around them. In an opposite corner was a man with his skull shattered and quite mad, who needed to be held down in bed, and in the next bed to the woman was a Frenchman dying of acute peritonitis. My friend was busy over in the theatre, whilst the faithful orderly and I attended to our ward.

The dying Frenchman was a man any woman might be proud of; his courage under acute pain was splendid. Towards dawn I asked him if I might write a letter to his wife. "No," he said, "soon I will be better and write myself." "But," I urged, "I want to write and tell her you are wounded. Give me just one message to send her."

Later on, when I saw that he was sinking, I said "Shall I call the Priest?" Then he knew what that implied, and the light went out of his eyes, whilst the good Curate silently prepared for him the Last Sacrament of the Church. It was not our rule to write to relatives of patients, there were too many, and time was short. But the courage of this man touched me, and I sat down by his still form and told her all I could, to make her strong to bear her grief. Later on I met her, but I will tell you of that presently.

Just about that time I gave the orphans a glorious party. We turned out our red-blanketed sitting-room and prepared all sorts of games. The toys we bought in Dunkerque were used for prizes, and the children themselves sang, recited and performed quite cleverly. It was a treat to see the poor little things enjoying so much merriment and having a good "tuck-in" of buns and sweets and other good things.

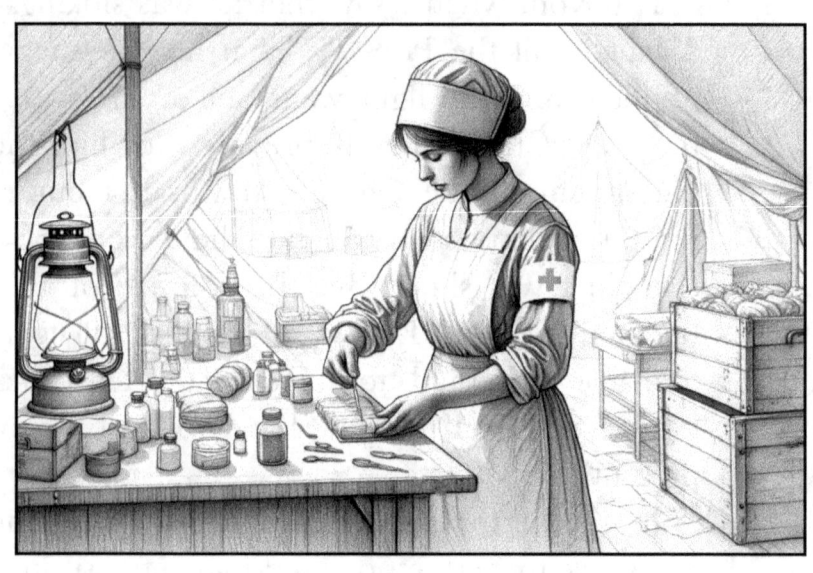

CHAPTER XII
THE BOMBARDMENT

WHEN our Field Hospital had been formed one of the privileges promised to all its members was that we should always be within sound and sight of the firing in the occupied trenches, and always situated about three or four miles behind the battle. The authorities never broke their word; in fact we added more than "sound and sight." The sensation of coming into "touch" with shot and shell was to be ours on more than one occasion, indeed at first we were more often on the spot where firing centred rather than four or five miles removed. We were now to go through our second bombardment, although, as you have seen, during our three months in Furnes we had been more or less bombarded all the time.

After Christmas the firing upon Furnes became incessant. There was hardly any peace and sleep was a luxury. The papers, so far as I know, rarely ever mentioned Furnes or the damage done there. Not because it was of no importance, but, on the contrary, because the King being there and it being Headquarters, it was too important to receive publicity. Towards the second week of January it was inadvisable to go on nursing the patients in the wards, and all who could be removed to safety were taken into France. We became just a dressing station and dumping ground for the dying or those who would die if they journeyed further, so the poor old Principal saw all his precious wine-cellars and vaults raided to make room for the wounded. We even had a theatre in a wine-vault, lit by candles and oil-lamps.

Scarcely had we removed the last patient into safety, and forbidden the staff to go up to their dormitory, when a great shell came crashing down, smashed through the dormitory roof and floor below, right into the empty ward, wrecking all that part of the building! Our Chief saw it was unwise to stay even in the cellars, so the ambulances were filled with patients and they were driven into Dunkerque. Some of the nurses were removed to La Panne and some to St. Malo near Dunkerque. They sought another hospital building elsewhere. All that time the town was under a hurricane bombardment. There was not a window left in Furnes. We had been told not to go outside, but one of our nurses, a Dutch girl, went round to her lodgings to fetch her hold-all. Crossing the market-place, a shell exploded near her, blowing her leg off from the hip. Although she received immediate attention nothing could save her. She bled to death. At a little cemetery in a village nearby we buried her, walking in procession behind the coffin.

It was during our stay at Dunkerque that a lady, swathed in crêpe veils and deep mourning, arrived. She was broken-hearted. We gathered between her sobs a confused history of a long journey of three or four days which she had taken from Lyons, suffering from cold and the disorganization of the railways. Arrived at Dunkerque she had been forbidden to travel further, as no civilians were allowed to go east of Dunkerque, which was in the war-zone of the armies. She was beside herself. If only she might look once on her husband's grave! Meanwhile she inquired for a certain Sister by name, and to my surprise it was my name she mentioned. In her hand was the letter I had written on Christmas night. It now seemed ages ago, for since then dozens of such cases had passed through my hands. It was all I could do to recall the individual facts. She longed for more details. How could I tell her of her loved one's sufferings? She wanted his last words, but he did not even realize he was dying. There was little it was possible to tell her, while as to his grave, in those early days it was difficult to find individual graves. Graves there were in plenty, by the hundreds and thousands, but which one?

We were just entering an ambulance on the eve of departure for our new hospital about twenty-five miles away. We were going to drive through Furnes to visit the brave doctors and students who insisted on staying in the College precincts to run the emergency dressing station. So, at the last minute, I bundled the poor widow in amongst us, unbeknown to the authorities, and we were shut in. At Furnes I got hold of a kind orderly, once a professor, and told him to show her a nice-looking grave to comfort her. She fell on my neck in a flood of tears, and that was the last I saw of her.

PART III

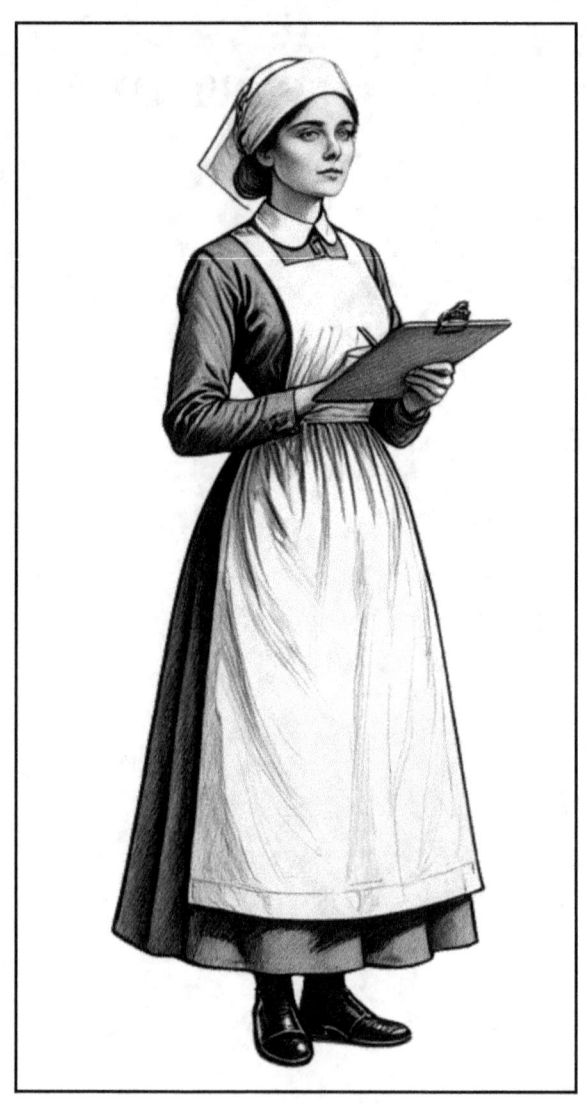

CHAPTER XIII
HOOGESTADT

OUR new hospital was at Hoogestadt. It was situated about seven or eight miles south of Furnes on the Ypres Road. This road ran parallel to the firing-line, about three or four miles to the west. We were about seven miles north of Ypres. The little hamlet of Hoogestadt straggled along the main road a mile to the north while south of us, the River Yser crossed the road, and just near there, in those early days, the British lines began. We had strict boundaries. We were not allowed to go farther than a certain village by the Yser to the south, nor were we allowed to go east of our hospital, the main road forming the boundary line. We might go as far as we liked into France. The almshouse which we new occupied had given up its residents. Our car removed nearly all the old bedridden men and women into France; one small corner still holding a few old men and women with some nuns to take care of them. It was a long two-story building with grounds in front. Behind were farm buildings and fields, sloping down to a brook. Opposite was a farm, in the grounds of which was a large convoy of Belgian ambulance cars under the charge of a young American.

The kitchen became our dining-room, our bedroom was up under the roof in a long attic which ran from one end of the great building to the other, with no partitions between. It was approached by a spiral staircase of fifty stairs. Here we all slept, about twenty-six nurses, thirty orderlies and kitchen staff, and six or seven Flemish laundry maids. We tied bandages from the rafters, pinning sheets to these, and so forming little rooms. Two nurses were allowed one tiny sky-light between them. Here we lived for ten months. A sugar case formed a dressing table. Later on we added the luxury of a zinc wash-tub, but circumstances were not conducive to personal cleanliness, hot water was precious and there were fifty stairs to carry it all up and down again. I don't remember that the place was ever swept or washed.

The chief feature outside was **MUD**, and a long straight road with trees on either side. Our front gateway was a Slough of Despond, likewise the farmyard behind. Our sanitary arrangements would not have passed the Health Boards at home. The farmyard was an interesting study in things ancient and modern---a mixture of peace and war.

Cows roamed around amongst motor ambulances and cars painted war-grey with huge red crosses upon them. Soldiers carried in stretchers of wounded or carried out the dead, nuns sat milking cows, infirm old almshouse women in large mob caps pottered about, while army nurses flew past on divers errands. Mechanics mended car machinery and rough ploughmen beat the corn with old-fashioned flails in the same barn. Around all was mud, mud, mud. A great cesspool ran under a large part of the farm yard quite close to the well---where the pump-handle squeaked day and night---from which we got all the drinking water.

Just about this time we had a new chef. Maurice had to return to the trenches. This new man had such an interesting career that he is worth mentioning. He too was another genial, sunny soul with a ready smile and a soft place in his heart for nurses.

He had been a prisoner under the Germans; and his skill as cook gave him a place with a great General at the Front. One night the Huns had taken a new city, so there was a dinner party. Our chef seasoned all the dishes with liqueurs; the sauces he flavoured with brandy, and he plied them with wine by the gallon. When he had succeeded in making all the gallant company thoroughly drank and the General lay under the table, he took up his hat and walked off! Escaping into Holland he was interned. There he obtained a post with a nobleman and was well paid. But, like the Jews in captivity, he sighed for his native land, so he forged a passport and, at a propitious moment when another banquet was under way, he went out on an errand and never returned. He preferred standing at our kitchen stove from 6.00 A. M. to 11.00 P. M., serving meals to two hundred people for practically no remuneration.

The next few pages are mostly about people, they are histories of heroes we nursed. For two months during that winter my friend and I were in charge of a small ward. We were only comfortably busy, as things were slack during the winter owing to the mud. Amongst the patients were four interesting cases who still write to us.

The first was Joseph. He was a dear boy, and stayed with us so long that we got to know him well. At Hoogestadt we nursed the Premier Division of the Belgian Army, and the Premier Guides were a body of cavalry in that Division. The officers formed the Royal Horse Guards stationed in peace times outside the Royal Palace at Brussels. We were stationed at the section where the Premier Guides fought and lived when out of the trenches. Joseph belonged to them. He came to us with a large wound in his leg. It pierced right through the calf, tearing the muscles from the shin-bone nearly all the way from the knee to the ankle. The doctors fixed it up, but very soon it went gangrenous. The surgeon said the only way to be sure of the mischief not spreading was to cut off his leg. I begged him to allow me to syringe it every half hour and meanwhile I removed him outside into the winter sunshine, fixing his leg up so that the air played all around the wound, and left it absolutely exposed all day long. It did well, and the gangrene came off in one big slough, leaving fresh, red flesh underneath.

He was outside at one meal hour, and I was busy in the ward behind him, when some one shouted out "Sister, quick! Joseph is bleeding to death!" I seized a tourniquet from a cupboard and rushed around, fixing it on. The surgeon who was called said there was now really nothing to be done but to take that leg off, as the main artery had sloughed through and the foot would get no circulation. Again I coaxed him to wait for a while and see if the foot really looked that way. We watched the leg anxiously the next few days. All the little veins and arteries took up the work of the big one, and the foot continued to thrive, likewise Joseph himself. His leg took a long time healing, and after he left us he went to a Paris hospital where he had all sorts of modern treatment for that torn muscle. But Joseph is now head mechanician in a large war motor works in France, with full use of both legs!

Eugene was in a bed next to him, and he owed his life to my friend's special care. He was about twenty-three years old, a married man with two children. From a photograph I should judge that he was handsome, but we never saw him at that stage. When he came in, there were grave doubts as to whether he could live. He had a hole in the back of his skull and his brains protruded. He was paralysed all down his right side, and quite helpless, for his left arm was broken in several places. Added to that he was literally "pelleted" all over face and body with small bits of shrapnel, cloth and mud being driven into each tiny wound. His face was badly swollen. You could not distinguish a feature, and he was caked in mud and blood. The skull was trephined and he lay unconscious for a good while. He needed constant attention, as both arms were useless. The left arm was set in splints and day by day little bits of shrapnel were dug out till we had cleaned up the whole surface of his body and cleared out the cloth and mud. He gradually got better, and he even began to get the use of his right leg before he left us. My friend often hears from him. Both legs are normal now, the bones in his left arm are set all right, some of his good looks have returned to him, and under special treatment he has got back the partial use of his right arm and is also being taught a new trade to support his family.

Ernst Handschutter is another most interesting case from a surgical point of view. He had a piece of shrapnel embedded in his heart. They cut, open his left breast, took out a piece of rib and exposed the heart to full view. Removing the outer skin of the heart, they found the bit of shrapnel, took it out, and sewed him up again. Afterwards Ernst's hands and feet looked rather blue and felt cold and clammy so some weeks later they opened him up again, and found a bit of skin had adhered to the heart and was impeding its proper beating. They loosened it and closed him all up for the second time. The operation this time was a complete success, and soon after Ernst was walking about. Now he is an orderly in a base hospital.

The fourth case I have kept until last. He is not only an almost unique surgical ease but a remarkable hero. Jean Lassoux is his name. He was a wholesale brush-maker from Liège, a man about thirty-seven. He was brought into our ward on a stretcher, with his head enswathed in blood-stained bandages. A bullet had gone through his left eye, damaged part of the brain and come out by the right ear. The surgeon said nothing could be done for him at present; he must just lie still, and the bandages which had been applied in the trench must not be touched. He was profoundly unconscious and breathed heavily. We thought that he was dying. As he lay there in that pitiful condition the Colonel of the regiment was announced, with other officers. Opening a little leather case, he took out the highest order of the Belgian Army, "The Premier Order of Leopold," pinned it on the wounded man's shirt, placing by him a long parchment on which were enrolled the name of his regiment, congratulations on his bravery, and records of a list of brave deeds which won him honour and distinction. Jean Lassoux had upon three occasions played a hero's part:

  1. When his Colonel asked for a volunteer to go over a hill and reconnoitre, at the grave risk of his life, as the Germans were on the other side of the hill, Jean offered and went.

  2. On two occasions in a burning town he rescued the occupants of a burning house; once, penetrating into the cellars with the fire blazing all around, and bringing up the suffocating refugees. Another time, climbing up a post when the first floor was in flames and the staircase burnt, he rescued the people upstairs.

  3. On the occasion of receiving his present head wound he had scrambled over the trench to a wounded comrade outside. Seizing the man's belt in his teeth, he crawled along low on the ground, carrying him, like a dog would, to a place of safety,

when he fell forward unconscious.

To return to his recovery in the ward, that first night he became exceedingly violent and noisy, so the night-nurse gave him a small dose of morphia. That nearly finished him. When we came on duty he was breathing three respirations a minute. We started on artificial-respiration and the treatment for opium poison. We worked him like a pump all that day, alternating the treatment by slapping him with scalding and ice-cold wet cloths. He came round and was very cross at our rough handling. Just then another man was dying in the next bed. We had to leave off and attend to him, and afterwards lay him out. By this time Jean had relapsed into the same torpor again. So we started the pump-handle business all over again. When we went off duty at eight P. M. we were rewarded by seeing a very cross Jean trying to get out of bed and go back to the trenches!

Jean was with us for weeks; his brain was not normal, even when he left us. During the first part of the time we held him in bed. His constant remarks were "Where are my boots? Where is my gun? I want to kill those damned Boches!" As he became clearer he was told that he never could go back to the trenches as he had only one eye, and was deaf in one ear. But he rejoined, "If I had two eyes I should shut one to look down my gun and shoot." He was so set on going back that, seeing the circumstances, the King granted him special leave to return. Since then he has served two years in the front line of trenches, been wounded and in hospital twice, but always returning to shoot "those damned Boches!" Jean was a gifted poet. He wrote many war poems. I did not think he would remember me because his brain was not quite clear, but months after he came back and gave me a hilarious greeting. Since then he has often written to me, his letters being sometimes in verse, all about his comrades and trench life.

The cold winter was passing. A body of soldier-workmen had built us a new front drive and filled up the Slough of Despond in our farmyard. The flooded Yser once more returned within the limits of its banks. Out in the fields little pink daisies grew among the grass, and down in a certain wood golden daffodils rejoiced our hearts and made the wards bright with spring. The country-side was covered with green buds and spring flowers. The everlasting mud had dried up. Preparations for a new offensive also were on foot, and every one felt that we were on the eve of great events. Who could believe, as we looked around the quiet country---fields being ploughed, birds building nests, larks soaring in the air---that the greatest war in history was being fought out, that Death and Desolation were blotting out Nature's beauty and depriving the world of the best of its manhood?

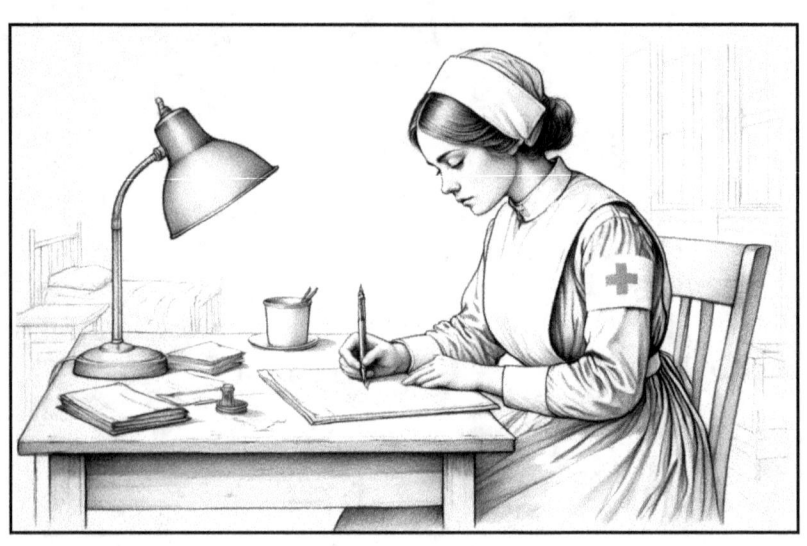

CHAPTER XIV
THE SECOND BATTLE OF YPRES

IN April, 1915, the operation theatre was put in my charge at night. Just myself and an orderly ran it. The orderly, Albert, was six feet, three inches high, and prided himself on two facts. First, that he bore the same name as his beloved Master, and second that he had been footman in the King's Palace. Of hospital work he was blissfully ignorant, and although he was my constant, willing helper in the time that followed, he learned everything by bitter experience---mine the bitterness, his the experience.

During the comfortless dull winter, with very little work to do, many of our surgeons and nurses had left us to join the English forces, where there lay promotion and remuneration. Also patriotism demanded our young doctors by now. We were thus reduced to three surgeons and nine nurses, the students having returned to London. Suddenly, one afternoon, about April 23rd, there was a long boom and roar all the way along the Front, from Nieuport in the extreme north to where the Ypres Salient bent round towards the south-west and vanished in the distance. After dark, magnesium-flares lit up the night, while the crackle of a million rifles and machine guns could be beard far away in the pauses of the artillery like water spluttering on a red hot stove.

My friend and I went out into the grounds and stood on a little mound watching the display. From the sea past Dixmude, Steenstraat, Ypres, round it swept in a half-circle, one blaze of flame and fire, while flashes and sudden bursts of light denoted huge explosions. The deafening roar of our guns could be heard to perfection in our long garret, whose sloping roof made an excellent sounding-board. Our ramshackle building rocked and swayed, shuddering from its foundations as in an earthquake. Blast after blast roared and belched forth, seemingly from under us. The laundry maids rushed shrieking down the stairs, thinking that the Germans were wiping us out of existence. Up till now none of us had had any idea that siege-guns lay hidden almost in our garden. Harmless-looking pig sties in the farms around sheltered the sinister muzzles of great guns; sunny springtime copses hid away under their branches giant siege-guns. We were really situated in the artillery-firing-line. Very soon we learnt to distinguish between the sound of shells sent from our guns and that of missiles travelling towards us from the German lines.

Our hospital soon became a shambles, the theatre a slaughter house. We started working that day, April 23rd, and we never stopped for about two weeks. Operations continued day and night, with two tables occupied all the time. A watchman controlled the ambulances as they swept round the drive and lined up one behind the other. Their bleeding loads were hurried into the building, and along the wide corridor that ran the length of the house was a double row of stretchers lying either side of the walls. Hundreds of minor cases were turned away to travel into France.

We received sixty-five cases that first night, and performed thirty operations! Every case was at Death's door. There lay British, Germans, French, Belgians, their greenish-grey faces looking ghastly in the dim light. Remember, we had only nine nurses for night and day work. There were only two of us on the ground floor, where there were two little wards and the theatre. We called some of the day nurses to help. If these men were to be saved it was only by immediate restoratives. We flew from man to man, inserting hypodermic-needles, giving saline-injections by the dozen. In the X-Ray department we were cutting off their clothes as they lay on the stretchers. Soon a mountain of clothes lay outside the back door---British, Belgian and German uniforms. Gas had been used in the trenches for the first time that day. There they lay, fully sensible, choking, suffocating, dying in horrible agonies. We did what we could, but the best treatment for such cases had yet to be discovered, and we felt almost powerless.

As to the theatre, one case was lifted off, a wet cloth mopped the blood on to the floor and another was lifted on. The good chauffeurs, who had been under fire collecting the wounded from the trench dressing-stations, made the journey several times in one night. Yet, weary as they were, they would seize a mop and pail and swill up some of the blood from the sloppy floor, or even hold a leg or arm while it was sawn off. I could do nothing but boil hundreds and hundreds of instruments over wretched petrol stoves that constantly got blocked and worked badly, and hand with the utmost rapidity to the surgeons working at both tables the instruments and cloths they needed to get on with their jobs. Huge abdominals, one after the other, trephining cases, amputations, ligaturing blood vessels in important places---on it went, those three surgeons never resting a minute for twenty-four hours on end. This continued from early that evening for two weeks. But the first night was the worst. Sixty-five cases was the number admitted. After that it varied from twenty-eight to fifty every night. Nearly all the cases travelled under cover of darkness so as to hide the Red Cross Ambulance from the Germans. That is why we were so hard pressed during the night. We found our staff hopelessly inadequate for its work as regards numbers. It was most difficult to procure English surgeons, as they were all needed in the British Army; also nurses could get any amount of good work in our own military hospitals now.

The Belgian military authorities soon solved the problem of surgeons by sending us a staff of Belgian Military surgeons with a Major at the head of it. This had its advantages and disadvantages. Our English surgeons did not like working under them at all; their methods were different, for one thing. The Belgian surgeons were very good to us nurses and really appreciated our work. The fact was they had now plenty of their own surgeons, trained in Belgian methods, but they had very few trained nurses. At first there was a great deal of misunderstanding between us, but things soon settled down and we worked very happily together.

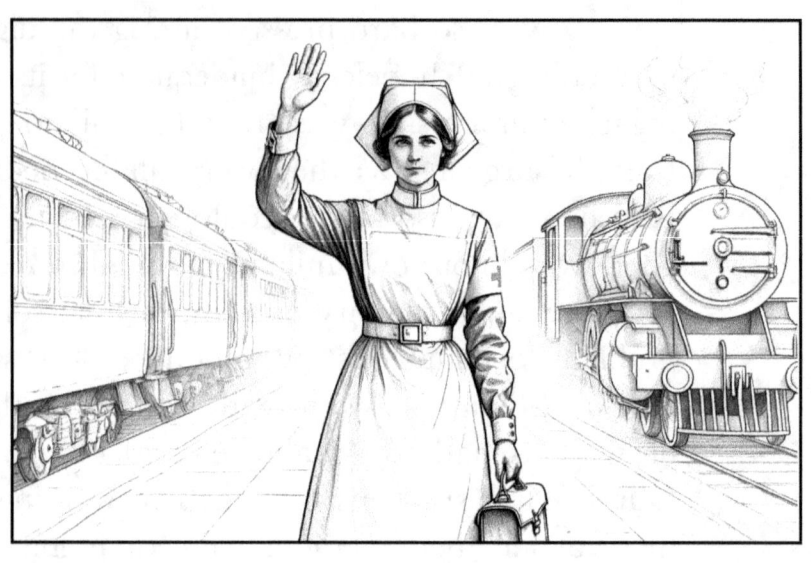

CHAPTER XV
A MILITARY HOSPITAL

WE were now a fully recognized Belgian Military Hospital although we were staffed by English surgeons and nurses. But the arrival of the Belgian Surgeon Major and his staff of officers gave us a standing we never had before, and a Power was behind us. After the great rush of April, 1915, we assumed more and more the nature of a base hospital, yet with the unspeakable advantage of being only three or four miles from the battle-line. We were thus able not only to save a great many lives that would have died during a long initial journey, but also to see our patients well on the road to recovery before we sent them, not to a base-hospital now, but to a convalescent home. We enlarged our borders and our boarders and added. four large wooden huts. These came out in sections from England, and it took twenty soldiers just one day to erect one hut. They were raised off the ground on wooden rests, held thirty beds each and had two little rooms at either end bathroom and lavatory one end, nurses' sitting room and kitchen the other. They were fitted with mica in lieu of glass windows.

A very interesting and necessary branch of our work was the X-Ray Department. We had possessed an X-Ray room ever since we had been at Hoogestadt, but it now sprang suddenly into fame, being reorganized by no less a person than the renowned Madame Curie, who discovered radium! For two or three weeks she lived with us, sharing our daily life, sitting next to us at meals, the most unassuming and gentlest of women. Her daughter was with us too, and stayed there all that summer after her mother left to aid other hospitals. They brought their own motor-ambulance which held the dynamo which worked the X-Ray apparatus. Madame Curie used to rise about five A. M., and have an early breakfast. As I was on night duty, it was my delight to set a table out in the garden and serve her breakfast myself. Often as we sat drinking a cup of coffee she would chat with me, taking a keen interest in all our work.

The summer heat now became as intense as the winter was cold. In our garret we suffered both extremes. In fact, when we slept during the day (on night duty) the sun poured down on that room so that it was like an oven. So my friend took to sleeping out in an open field with a large Japanese parasol tied at the head of the bed. I have often seen her lying there fast asleep, with a cow munching round the sides of the bed! So I sent home for a tent, and we slept in that. Often on sunny afternoons I have lain awake, gazing up through the aperture watching the airplanes buzzing past overhead, or seeing a Taube sail up from the east, whilst a sharp contest ensued, the shrapnel exploding all around like little balls of cotton wool. German and Ally airplanes were so common now that we never took any notice of them, excepting when we all once ran out to watch a German plane falling to earth, a mass of flames. It dropped behind Dixmude, and I still have a piece of a wing. On another occasion three Taubes hovered over our hospital for half an hour or more. We expected every moment to see the place come down in ruins, but evidently he decided we were not a hospital and so would not waste his shells on us.

Now that gas had made its appearance and come to stay, we supplied our patients with respirators soaked in hyposulphate. These we placed in little mackintosh bags at the head of each bed. We also each carried one in our own pockets. Every one who has followed the papers knows all about that awful time in the spring of 1915, round about Ypres. The aftermath I have already described as we experienced it in our theatre and wards. So near were the Germans to breaking through just where we were that all arrangements had been made for our hurried flight. The young American on the farm opposite was to help us. First the wounded were to go in the ambulances, then as many nurses as could he accommodated; lastly the orderlies and men of our staff were to escape on foot. But, thank goodness, the Germans never have broken through. It is we now who are playing that little game.

The soldier-workman had not only mended the road and front approach, but had planted flower beds, and now our front garden became a great feature in our life. Three times a week a band played to the patients, beds were brought out in the shade of the trees, whilst officers and soldiers visited their wounded friends. Meals were served outside to them, and the staff had a long table under the trees where we took our meals. Round at the back were the huts where we often had entertainments. Bands of soldiers, during their repose from the trenches, gave concerts, boxing and wrestling matches, juggling and all sorts of entertainments for the wounded men.

We had our share of pleasant, times. Near to us was one of the Allies' captive balloons. These, great pumpkin-shaped things are placed every mile or so all along the back of our lines, as the eyes of the army. The one nearby had been a source of great danger to us at one time. It floated up just over our heads and the Germans constantly shelled it, never hitting it, but the shells came down in our premises and two farms near us were injured.

A party of soldiers eating their meal in the farmyard were all wounded and killed. We sent a petition to have the balloon moved farther away, so it was placed higher up the road. Major Gerard was in charge of it, with about fifty men. These men were not very busy, so they had time on their hands. They were a most gifted set. They all lived in a barn and this barn they turned into a theatre, built a fine stage with all the scenery, painted screens and drop-curtain, made stage furniture, etc. They wrote plays, made all the actors' clothes and acted the plays as well. The hay was piled up tier above tier, opposite the stage, for the audience, and two front rows of seats formed the stalls. In the well in front the band played. Here we witnessed the most thrilling pieces ever produced at any theatre, and heard barrack-room concerts! It was well for us that our knowledge of the French language was limited, and that we did not understand all the subtleties of their humour and slang! From my seat in the hay I have peeped through the boards across the plain where the sky was red with the battle, and in between the band-playing heard the boom of the cannon.

Another pastime which we enjoyed that summer

was riding. In a previous chapter I spoke of the Premier Guides Officers. These men, before they donned khaki, were a picturesque body of cavalry. They wore crimson riding breeches, bottle green tunics and gay little red forage caps with swinging gold tassels set at a rakish angle on the side of the head. They all belonged to the Belgian nobility, and most of them once possessed old chateaux now desecrated by German troops. Their riding is well known in sporting circles; they are among the champion horsemen of the world, having taken prizes at the Olympia Horse Show and shaken hands with King George of England. Their horses were superb, some of them worth £1000 or more. We had nursed some of these men, and to show their gratitude three or four times they invited us out riding. One occasion lives in my memory always. It was Springtime, before the April rush. They invited us over to the seaside village of Bray-Dune, among the sandhills. We went in one of our ambulances, seven of us. Arriving at an inn, they had, prepared for us a champagne-luncheon. After lunch fourteen lovely horses were led up by orderlies and we mounted. Then we flew over the short turf, dunes and sandy valleys for miles and miles. At one place they had prepared trenches, barriers and ditches for us to jump, while nearby was a sand cliff about fifty feet high, almost perpendicular. After galloping up the sloping approach, the horses put all four feet together, leaned back on their haunches, and so slid down this cliff! It was perfect riding, for they never indulged in any monkey-tricks. Then, clearing the bank on to the seashore and finding it low tide, we raced over the firm wet sand for several miles back to Bray-Dune.

Upon another occasion we went for a luncheon party, at the Farm where their Colonel and Major were quartered. The walls were decorated with startling pictures from periodicals of young ladies in bathing costumes, etc. We walked around the picture-gallery, the old Colonel explaining to us that the choicest works of art were missing, as he had sent his young Lieutenant round previous to our arrival to censor and excise the more advanced artistic productions! We invited them back to afternoon tea in our tree-shaded garden, and once we even had a dinner party out there by the moonlight in their honour.

Nearby was a farm which was the headquarters of the Blue-Cross. Here all the wounded and convalescent horses were attended, under the charge of Lieutenant H-----. Many of these horses were well again and fit to ride. Lieutenant H----- turned his place into a regular riding-school and taught many of the Sisters to ride, taking us out in parties when off duty. We went long expeditions into France by little unfrequented lanes. It was he who initiated us into the fearsome joys of a military "charge." We just gave the horses rein, and they went, like a shot out of a bow. It was like sailing through the air on an airplane, with a thunder of hoofs and cloud of dust taking the place of the roar of the engines and the smoke of guns. During that summer we had two surgeons with us, friends of mine from the East. Often we rose early and rode before duty, from 6:00 to 8:00 A. M. We were very naughty about disobeying rules, we used to wander out-of-bounds to the east of us, all among the troops, exploring towards the battle-line. The best of it was the Belgians thought the doctors were British officers, as they wore khaki, and instead of asking for passports they saluted us! Sometimes, just two of us nurses went off alone, or even singly, following the little narrow footpaths among the cornfields for miles and miles; or, when the crops were gathered, galloping across country. Twice my horse bolted, and once a shying pony named Koko threw me, and I returned home in one of our ambulances, stunned, and with a dislocated thumb. But I was on duty again next day.

About midsummer we were moved to the Officers' Ward, which was a new departure. Formerly the officers had been nursed with the soldiers, but now the soldiers were moved into the huts outside, and the main building was used only for the large staff. There were a theatre, X-ray rooms, receiving room (where the newly arrived wounded were examined), offices, kitchens, and just one small ward of eight beds for the officers My friend and I were put in charge, one on night and one on day-duty and there we made some very good friends whom we have since met in London when they had leave or were convalescent. Once we had a Belgian captain of an airplane, who fell three thousand metres and only fractured his shoulder-blade! We tried to give these men something of the comforts they would have had in a London hospital. Oh, the letters I wrote to Red Cross sewing parties! And the handsome harvest we received to reward my literary labours! Crates upon crates of lovely pyjamas, socks, bed linen, and even fancy tray-cloths. We made our ward a most attractive place, and tried to make up to those poor fellows for having no home or friends, but only miserable thoughts of their home-folk under German rule.

The officers shared the same food as the staff and had evening-dinner. We used to bring a little table from the ward outside our windows into the front garden, and with our two orderlies to wait on us we used to dine by moonlight with those patients who were able to walk. Once or twice they came riding with us, and one of them, a Premier Guides officer, was taken to England by my friend, C----- to convalesce at her own home, where she motored him all over our lovely country and managed to have a very good time!

Our hospital was now top-hole. We had every appliance and arrangement that could make for the well-being of a modern war-hospital. The military saw to it that we were well supplied with soldiers to do all the work, and our home-society now paid the nurses' salaries, so we had a plentiful supply of help. The long road outside saw a constant stream of British cars bringing in wounded and taking them on to France. This road, with its little straw sentry-boxes placed every mile or so along it, with sentries standing at attention and shouting for the password to every motorcar, was one of the busiest thoroughfares in Europe. It was quite straight, vanishing over the horizon in both directions, with trees, denuded of their lower branches, meeting overhead. Here artillery, motor lorries, troops of British and Belgian soldiers, little convoys of "mitrailleuses," consisting of machine-guns mounted on tiny cars, each pulled by two handsome trained dogs (beautiful, intelligent creatures led by their own kind soldier), Red Cross ambulances, general staff cars, and, last but not least, every now and then, bodies of grey uniformed, closely cropped German prisoners, surrounded by Arab cavalry or

Belgian guards, marched stolidly on.

Often this same road was the scene of a slow, sad procession, which, leaving our gates, headed by an ambulance draped with the Allied flags, and followed by the curé, some orderlies and sometimes nurses, walked slowly up the road to a little plot of ground, owned by us, in the midst of the cornfields, whose crop was little crosses. Never shall I forget the funeral of some gassed British soldiers who died at our place. We placed them side by side in our Red Cross ambulances, draped with the Union Jack, and all our doctors and nurses in uniform walked slowly behind them to their last resting-place.

We were honoured by many visits from King Albert and Queen Elizabeth. Her Majesty used to walk around the wards, preceded by officers carrying piles of cigarettes, chocolates and flowers for the soldiers. She was always very simply dressed and her manners were equally simple. Stopping at each bed she chatted with the men, inquiring all about their circumstances.

During that summer the Canadians put in an appearance near us. There were five hundred quartered on two farms; and at first they were busy laying concrete-foundations for siege-guns outside Dixmude. They soon discovered us and we became great friends. We had other visitors also; people of repute from England and other countries came on tour, visiting us on the way. Naval officers from the coast, also personal friends in the British lines stationed at Ypres, Poperinghe and elsewhere, rode over.

This history will not be complete without telling you about my General. I call him mine, because I had the honour of being his special-nurse on day-duty. He was the General of the Premier Belgian Division, therefore a personage of great importance. He was also a great friend of the King Albert, who sent him his own bed and mattress because he found ours hard! One evening he came in on a stretcher, and was placed on a bed in the Officers' Ward. He was a man of about sixty-five years of age, seriously wounded in the lower part of the back, his hip bones being badly shot away and the flesh laid open down to the spine. All the officers were quickly moved into a hut, grumbling and protesting at being turned out of their own little corner and leaving their own attendants, while the now large empty room was transformed into a pleasant living-room. We sent over to Furnes for the old priest's best carpet and some upholstered chairs, and arranged gay screens around. Madame Curie fixed up for the General an electric-bell worked from her dynamo, and a telephone communicating with Headquarters by his bedside. Her Majesty sent quantities of lovely flowers, and we made that room like a first-class nursing-home apartment. Not that the dear old General wanted it, he was a regular Spartan, a born soldier, and used to the simplest mode of living. So long as his orders were obeyed promptly and to the letter and his bell answered on the moment, all went well; he asked nothing more. To me he showed an old-world courtesy, never allowing me to do anything he considered infradig, but insisting on my calling the orderly. His morning dressing was a solemn ceremony, needing about an hour's preparation. The Major, Lieutenants and British surgeons were all summoned to be present at the function, while the Major performed it.

There were other ceremonies which took place in the General's room. General Joffre arrived one day and decorated him with the Legion of Honour. After Joffre had pinned the medal on his breast and kissed him on both cheeks he came over and talked to me for a few minutes about the General's progress. Another day King Albert arrived and gave him a medal, one only given to high officers, ---the Order of the Cross. A certain great man, a member of the British Royal Family, was also deputed to be the bearer of the Victoria Cross from our King. Many great statesmen of Belgium and famous warriors of the Allies visited my General at one time or another.

It was autumn now. Sometimes in the afternoon

we wandered across the fields, picking blackberries which I made into pies or stewed for my illustrious patient. I spent a good part of my time trying to concoct little dainties for him, and bothering the chauffeur, who bought our stores each day in Dunkerque, to search the shops for some new delicacy. In those rambles we strolled along the banks of little brooks where forget-me-nots fringed the edges, passed through farmyards where nuns in their quaint costumes sat on three-legged stools milking cows, and soldiers leaned over the gates laughing and chatting. By-and-by the sun sank, a ball of fire, while mist rose like a veil from the low flat country. In the glow of the glorious sunset airplanes chased each other overhead, little puffs of smoke dotted the clear blue sky, whilst the bark of guns and the reports of explosions overhead all played a weird part in the rural evening scene. Birds chirped in the hedges where we gathered blackberries, while on the horizon the roar of artillery formed the bass of the orchestra. The General progressed rapidly. In a month he was able to dispense with my services. Soon the morning came when I entered his room to bid him farewell. Handing me an immense bouquet, he kissed me on both cheeks in approved French fashion. Then we climbed the car and were off to Calais, en route for England, waving regretful good-byes to white-capped groups of nurses and our dear Belgian friends.

It was at the Calais station, while we were lunching, that I noticed other travellers give furtive glances through the windows. Wondering what excited their curiosity, I rose. Just outside, in a little group of three, engaged in the discussion of weighty matters, stood Lord Kitchener, General Joffre, and Mr. Balfour. It was my first and last view of England's military idol. Before the historic figure of that Great Warrior I will drop the curtain, for this seems a fitting conclusion to thirteen months' life at the Back of the Front.

I left Belgium October 5th, 1915.

www.ingramcontent.com/pod-product-compliance
Lightning Source LLC
Chambersburg PA
CBHW052057070526
44584CB00017B/2223